An E
In America

Richard F. Morton, M.D.

FRASER PUBLISHING COMPANY
Burlington, Vermont

Copyright © 1997 by Richard F. Morton

Published in 1997 by Fraser Publishing Company
          a division of
          Fraser Management Associates, Inc.
          Box 494
          Burlington, Vermont 05402
          800-253-0900

All rights reserved. No part of this book may be reproduced or transmitted in any form or by any means, electronic or mechanical, including photocopying, recording, or by any information storage and retrieval system, without permission in writing from the publisher, except in the case of brief quotations to be used in critical reviews or articles.

Library of Congress Cataloging-in-Publication Data
Morton, Richard F., 1924-
    An English doctor in America / Richard F. Morton.
      p.   cm.
    ISBN 0-87034-127-8 (alk. paper)
    1. Morton, Richard F., 1924-   . 2. Obstetricians—United States—Biography
    3. Obstetricians—England—Biography. 4. Obstetrics—Anecdotes. I. Title.
    RG510.M67A3   1997
    610'.92—dc21
    [b]
                                                       97-20252
                                                           CIP

Printed in the United States of America

Contents

Chapter 1
Christmas in Montana 1

Chapter 2
Antecedents 7

Chapter 3
Indoctrination 23

Chapter 4
Under the Dome 65

Chapter 5
In the Shadow of Ebetts Field 91

Chapter 6
Young Man Goes West 109

Chapter 7
Indian Heaven 121

ACKNOWLEDGEMENTS

The author is indebted to three people, without whose assistance this book would not exist. They are, Belle Magram, who deciphered my handwriting and typed the manuscript; Suzanne Erfurth, who expertly edited the work and Kate, my wife who despite the invasion of her privacy assisted and encouraged me from the beginning to the end.

INTRODUCTION

All my friends (er, both of them actually) implored me to write this book. They sought immunity from listening to any more of my stories, reasoning that recording them would cure me forever from recounting others. They were correct.

Writing one's memoirs has been termed the last act of self-promotion, a definition with which I have no quarrel and, I suspect, neither will my readers.

Chapter 1

Christmas in Montana

It was snowing on Christmas Eve in Spokane as I boarded the train, seated high in the leading dome car. Our route lay first along the valley beside the river, then we crossed into Idaho, where the scenery became rugged and mountainous. The train slowed as the track climbed, twisting and turning, the great light from the locomotive illuminating the way. The snowflakes, thicker now, glistened in our light, twirling as they fell and drifting away among the pines.

Arriving in Libby, a small logging town bisected by a fast-flowing river, I was met by my host, Doctor Bob Campbell, the local G.P. His house, built of wood, looked down on the river and over the town to the mountains beyond. It was full of my hosts' four children, a Labrador and two cats. A Christmas tree, gifts and a log fire made the Yuletide atmosphere complete.

Later, I was roused from a deep sleep by my hostess, asking me to join Bob at the hospital, where he faced a difficult delivery. I dressed, half awake, and received some directions. In their cold car I slid downhill to cross the river and drive through the strange deserted town, now deep in snow, to a small hospital.

It was 3:00 AM by the delivery room clock on Christmas Day, 1956. Bob was seated on the stool, his brow covered in sweat, his gown splashed with blood, his smile forced. A large woman was lying in stirrups on the table, semiconscious, undelivered. She was bleeding, not a flow but slowly and steadily, adding to the growing pool in the bucket. There was an I.V. drip running with clear fluid. In the basin were two pairs of discarded forceps. An anxious, tired nurse was the only other person in the room.

"I have been trying for nearly an hour," said Bob. "Her previous two were difficult but not as bad as this. I think it's bigger."

I asked the nurse where the anesthetist was.

"She's in Salt Lake, visiting her sister."

"I gave her some drip ether on a mask," added Bob. I inquired about blood supplies. The nurse informed me that they relied on volunteers and there was no blood available in the hospital. I then palpated the patient's belly and did a pelvic exam. She had a large baby presenting by the head, which had gotten through the pelvic inlet. The contractions were moderate and the nurse said they were weakening. I listened to the fetal heart, 105 and regular, and took the mother's blood pressure and pulse.

As I scrubbed, the term "treacherous multipara" flitted into my mind, an obstetrician's saying which refers to a woman who has delivered one or usually two babies vaginally, apparently without complication, and then has a larger one. Labor advances enough to deceive you into thinking she'll come through vaginally again, then descent stops, with the head stuck in the mid-pelvis. I thought, "She has deep transverse arrest." This means the head has not turned correctly to negotiate the narrowest part of the pelvis where two bony spines project, and further descent is impossible.

I knew the safest course for the baby, to avoid brain damage or death, was to deliver the mother by cesarean section. I could give a local anesthetic but that would not provide enough relaxation. Even if we could reposition her so I could give a spinal, her blood pressure would drop and she might go into shock. She needed a general anesthetic for a section, but even if we could locate an anesthetist an hour would have elapsed. If I imposed a section after an hour's delay and more bleeding, she would die.

I knew where the bleeding was coming from. She had cervical tears and vaginal lacerations as a consequence of the failed forceps attempts. I must deliver her vaginally and hope the baby survived. I recalled a saying by one of my English teachers, "If the Almighty can get the head into the pelvis, I, Leslie Williams, can get it out." These garbled thoughts were in my head as I scrubbed, and I reached a decision faster than my explanation can be read.

Gowned and gloved, I took Bob's place on the stool, and slipped my index finger into the birth canal feeling round the baby's head for an ear. I could just reach one, and by flipping it forward I could tell which way the head was facing, to the patient's right or left. The narrowest diameter of a baby's head is between the ears. In order to pass the spines of the mid-pelvis, the head must present that diameter to the passage. But this baby's head was ninety degrees out of alignment—therefore I had to turn it through a right angle and in the correct direction. To move the head, I had first to dislodge it, pushing it back up from the mid-pelvis in order to secure room to turn it. Using my left hand, I pushed the head up, gently, between contractions, when the uterus was lax. This was dangerous, for the umbilical cord can slip down in advance of the head, get squashed and asphyxiate the baby. I steadied the head and felt around. Good; no cord. Then I took in my right hand one half of a pair of Kielland's forceps with long, delicate sculpted blades used for turning, and sneaked it in alongside the baby's skull. Holding it steady, I inserted the companion blade on the other side.

These forceps have a sliding lock, permitting an uneven application, one blade further in than the other. But this time the lock closed easily in the middle of the slide, a sign of a good application—now I had the baby's head grasped by the blades. I knew, from the ear trick, which way to turn them so that the head presented as nature intended, and would, I hoped, pass the narrow space between the bony spines of the mid-pelvis. I turned the blades the requisite ninety degrees in the correct direction. To my satisfaction, the head turned also—the blades did not slip round the skull without turning it, which is what happens with an incorrect application.

Now I had to pull the head down through the mid-pelvis and deliver it, but this cannot be done with the turning blades. I grasped one of the heavy, solid, curved blades used for traction and slowly slipped off the light blade, replacing it with the heavy one, which had to be inserted carefully high into the pelvis to reach the baby's head. I repeated this with the second blade and the application felt secure.

I pulled gently, then rested, then pulled, and the head passed the mid-pelvis, moving down towards the roomier outlet. I continued to pull and rest, trying to stay in time with the contractions. Finally, a large head appeared, looking as if it had been three rounds with Rocky Marciano.

Bob suctioned the baby's mouth and throat while I prepared to deliver the shoulders. A big head means big shoulders and I did not want to get them held up. I told the nurse to push down on the mother's belly, whereupon one shoulder delivered. By reaching under the baby's head, I dislodged the other. Then, placing my hands on the baby's shoulders, I pulled downward, delivering a large boy whom I handed to Bob, who resuscitated him. The placenta delivered easily and, placing one of the large forcep blades as a retractor on the vaginal wall and asking the nurse to hold it, I inspected the birth canal. Blood was coming from tears on the cervix but I could see them and sutured them. Further bleeding came from the vaginal wall, which I repaired. If I haven't ruptured the uterus, I thought, maybe I have gotten away with this.

But when I stood and inspected the patient, I was alarmed; she looked, and her vital signs corroborated, bled out. "What's her blood group?" I asked the R.N.

"A-Pos.," she replied.

Bob spoke up: "I'm A-Pos. Draw a bottle from me quickly and transfuse her."

"I'll draw it," said the nurse, and she took Bob, a big man, to the X-ray room to lay him on the large table there, while I remained with the patient. I put a catheter into her bladder and wondered whether to pack the vagina. Obstetricians were divided into packers and non-packers and I veered to the latter group. If she was going to bleed again, I wanted to know it early, not let her soak a large pack first.

I was nervous about lowering her legs from the stirrups, as much of the blood had drained from them due to gravity. If they were lowered rapidly now, more blood would accumulate in them—in effect a further blood loss that she could not tolerate, and she would go into shock. So, using large elastic bandages, I wrapped her legs tightly, starting with the toes and ending with her groin, then I lowered them. I slid off her sweat-soaked gown and wrapped her in warm blankets, bathed her face and dried her hair. But we needed the blood, where was it?

Reaching the x-ray room, I found that the nurse had drawn the blood quickly but Bob had responded by vomiting and collapsing. She had started an I.V. on him. I strapped him on the table and left him, taking his blood and transfusing the patient. The nurse returned to monitor the baby and I remained with the patient and the debris in the delivery room. While the nurse checked on Bob, I used the time to record what had occurred.

The patient stabilized and I felt confident to move her to the ward as her bleeding appeared to have ceased. Bob gave a guarded prognosis for the baby, but he had not deteriorated. When the mother's and baby's charts were completed, we stepped out into the frigid air of predawn. There was a glimmer of light in the east as we drove home, Bob in the lead as I followed in the second car. After a blessed sleep, we returned around midday and found our patients improving.

On the day of my departure, I visited the mother, now almost recovered. Bob introduced me: "This is Professor Morton, a specialist from New York. Without his skill you and your baby would have died. You should feel grateful." (Another baby to be named Richard, I thought, but the first in Montana.)

"Should I?" she replied with spirit. "Before he meddled with me, I never had any problems—and don't you send me a bill," she shouted at me, "because I won't pay it!"

Chapter 2

Antecedents

On September 3, 1939, when World War II began, I was a pupil in Dulwich College, a boarding school in London, facing two years until graduation. All the boys welcomed the war, believing that it would enliven our sequestered, regulated lives. We were not disappointed. Bombs fell in the neighborhood, resulting in our evacuation to Kent, thirty miles south, where we intruders shared the premises at a smaller school. We started a war of our own and, over a thousand strong, were victorious over the local forces. Before we could consolidate our gains the bombing ceased, and we returned abruptly to London.

In wartime, chaos reigned, change was the norm, and life was speeded up. I benefited from these upheavals, for my experience during wartime subsequently launched me on a journey to America which I otherwise would not have taken.

My brother, six years my junior, and I lived fifteen miles south of London. Early in the war our neighbors' house was destroyed by a bomb, leaving nothing but a large hole in which blue flames burned. (They were away, and we were safe in a bomb shelter in the garden.) Many families were moving out of London, but Father was contrary and moved in, buying a home in Wimbledon, six miles from the city. Adjacent to the Common, it was a fine site which, in normal times, we would not have been able to afford. He explained that if Germany won it would make little difference where we lived, but if we won then Wimbledon would remain a desirable address, and so it proved.

Father had left school at sixteen, and worked in the Central London Post Office, Mount Pleasant, as a sorter. To augment his income he enlisted in the Territorial Army (National Guard), with the result that he was in the trenches at Flanders before Christmas 1914. He had married in August of that year on the outbreak of the Great War. He was one of only three men in his regiment of the London Rifle Brigade to survive until the Armistice in November 1918. He ascribed his escape to two factors: his refusal to accept promotion beyond that to Lance Corporal, and the protection given him, a Lewis machine gunner, by his comrades, who knew that if the gun was silenced their position would be overrun. Mother, devout, believed his deliverance was due to a miracle. His survival gave rise to a saying, "the Morton Luck." My brother and I have also been its beneficiaries. Only after his death did we find, hidden in his desk, the Military Medal and citation for valor in the field.

I saw little of Father when I was young, since he caught the 6:00 AM train to London and returned late. He retired in 1934 when I was ten, and we got to know one another. He was reserved, a pragmatist and atheist, showing little emotion, but he had one surprising characteristic. He was a humorist—spontaneously, genuinely funny. His humor was not cruel, and often self-deprecatory. He was well-informed, invariably correct on factual matters, but he abhorred pomposity and was quick to prick it, and he cared nothing for appearance, rank, or station.

Mother was the eldest of nine siblings, from a family in cockney London, where her mother ran a neighborhood store. This store was packed with goods, in sacks, barrels, tins, and jars, and items hung from the ceiling and flowed onto the pavement. Grandma knew her customers and where every item was. She lived to be 102, spending her last decade living with us in Wimbledon, where she continued to play the piano. (When I returned home after a long absence and bent down to kiss her she whispered, "They've forgotten to collect me.")

Mother had left school at twelve, but was gifted with a fertile imagination. My earliest memories are of her telling me stories while I rode in a pram. Once, we passed a goat tethered on a hillside by the railroad track. Mother told me of the goat's hopes, its pleasures and sorrows. We stopped by a store in whose window stood a large, colored rocking horse. She invented tales of the horse's exciting past and how he finally came to live in the shop. The Lyle's Golden Syrup tin had then, and does now, an enigmatic illustration of a lion lying down surrounded by swarming bees, and a legend, "Out of the strong came forth sweetness." Mother told me of the lion's past and how he came to his present predicament.

She wrote expressive letters to me weekly well into her nineties. On a visit to Wimbledon with our daughter Nancy, then four, we three walked on the Common and reached a large, lone tree. Nancy, ever dutiful, asked, "Grandma, may I climb that tree?" Mother replied, "We must ask the tree," and stood under it, apparently communing with it, then pronounced: "The tree says, 'I have many strong branches to bear you, leaves to shade you, and I am lonely. A little girl to climb and rest in my arms would be lovely, come, climb me.'"

In June 1941 our science teacher had good news. People were needed to work with radar, which was essential to detect enemy aircraft and vessels. Those proficient in physics were eligible for a two-year scholarship leading to a university degree. The school recommended me, I sat an examination, and I was admitted to London University in the Imperial College of Science. I spent the first three months living at home in Wimbledon, commuting to Kensington daily by subway.

I had led a sheltered life, never meeting anyone from a different background. This changed, because suddenly my class was transferred to Exeter, 170 miles away in the southwest peninsula, where a college, affiliated with London University, had been established. My roommate, the son of a Welsh coal miner, was more gifted than I, particularly in mathematics, which he taught me. (I reciprocated by teaching him bridge.) Our classes were small and informal, teachers were accessible, and learning ensued.

Early in 1943, following twenty enjoyable months, the time arrived to repay the education vouchsafed me. A few top students, including my roommate, were directed into research as civilians, and the majority of us were consigned to the military. Faced by the RAF's selection board I received some sound advice: "Say anything but make it short." Their first question was, "Why do you want to join the RAF?" "Sir, to shoot the Germans down." This exchange concluded the interview. The truth was that the RAF was attractive because the Navy was closed and the grim alternative was the Army. Ineligible for aircrew, I was designated for a technical job.

My introduction to basic training was inauspicious. I have large feet, size 13, thereby getting a good grip of the ground. To be kitted out, we were lined up in order of shoe size, small first. Standing barely six feet, weighing about 220 lbs., I was a dwarf among the giants at the end of the line. My boots fitted but only I knew that. With my hat sitting on my ears, my greatcoat trailing the ground, and my long, baggy trousers, I fell far short of the crisp silhouette espoused by the military.

My bedmate, lower bunk, was a cockney philosopher, incredibly old, over forty. Watching me write a letter to my mother, he admonished: "Your best friend in life isn't your mother, it's your bank account." I was miserable and showed it. "Cheer up mate, you'll soon be dead," declared my companion. Squads of recruits were dispatched at odd times. In the small hours a sergeant clumped into our hut, shone a flashlight into the lower bunk and bawled: "Are you draft?" "No mate, bottled," came the prompt reply.

Soon I was transferred to Officers Training School for six weeks' drilling. The RAF was not noted for discipline but what there was of it was most evident at large bases, with much shouting and saluting. At the operational level of a squadron airfield, where there was a job to be done, a more relaxed atmosphere prevailed.

I learned one valuable lesson while training. A warrant officer—who also could put more contempt into the word "gentlemen" than seemed possible—taught us how to give orders; namely, clearly. He warned us that before presuming an order had been ignored or disobeyed we must first ascertain that the recipient had understood it. He provided an illustration. He had been called to the canteen where a drunken airman, dancing on a table, was causing a commotion. Our instructor gave an order: "Airman, get down off that table." "Fuck you and fuck this table," the airman replied, whereupon he knew his order had been understood.

Upon graduation, resplendent in a new uniform as a wingless wonder, I was sent to a large base fifty miles north of London. In the officers' mess arose a peculiarly British crisis. Joe Louis, Master Sergeant and the world heavyweight boxing champion, was to give an exhibition. Should he be permitted into the officers' mess? This knotty problem was solved when two US staff cars arrived and Louis emerged and strolled into the mess, where he was enthusiastically received. Later, the Commandant, a small, officious man, unwisely decided he would introduce Louis from the ring. As he approached the champion, a voice rang out, "Hit him, Joe."

I was dispatched to an airfield in Lincolnshire, home to two squadrons of Lancaster bombers. My designation as an armament officer came as a surprise, for I was expecting duty in radar or signals. I had no engineering knowledge or aptitude, which was immediately recognized by the flight sergeants. However, the NCOs were impeded by reports and forms that had to be completed and returned to higher authority, and here I could make a contribution. I understood that the secret of success in military form completion lay in answering every question and filling in every line and box. The content of responses appeared irrelevant. I accordingly used "not applicable," "pending," "undetermined," "to be arranged," "forthcoming," "immaterial," "arbitrary," "imminent," "deferred," and other empty phrases in response to different questions. If the query demanded several responses such as 9a, 9b, 9c, I replied "see 5c," "ref 3d," "as in 4e."

The USAAF was bombing Germany by day, the RAF by night. American aircraft landed at our base because they were lost, which was not infrequent or surprising. England is diminutive in comparison to the United States. Our region, flat and close to the enemy coast, was packed with airfields, which looked alike from the air. Our weather, changeable and unpredictable, contributed to the confusion.

We were instructed to fraternize with our American cousins, which was easy, for they were likable, relaxed, and friendly. One visit remains memorable as it provided a real opportunity to fraternize. Instead of the usual B-17s, some Dakotas landed in the late afternoon, disgorging over a hundred U.S. nurses. All officers, all female, they burst into the mess, filling it with laughter, chatter, fragrance and energy. Their uniforms, tightly fitting, were covered with bars, stars, medals and colorful insignia. They were fresh from the States, adventurous, spontaneous, pulsating, eager. We were overwhelmed initially but recovered quickly.

The meteorological officer closed the airfield, citing sudden "poor weather." The adjutant decreed our visitors should sleep in the mess, and an equivalent number of junior officers were instructed to make alternative arrangements. Catering was inveigled to prepare a fine dinner. Flattery persuaded the camp band to play for dancing. Volunteer waiters appeared by magic. The chaplain agreed to deliver an invocation before dinner, believing this to be an American custom that would make the nurses feel at home. Following dinner the COs exchanged compliments, toasts were drunk and dancing began. This delightful evening was a fusion of the old world and the new, come again to our succour.

The American and British Air Forces had bombsights of differing designs. Each believed theirs superior. The result was that someone proposed that liaison might offer mutual benefits. To my surprise I was seconded, for two months, to a USAAF base to explore this proposition with an American colleague. My immersion into American culture was congenial. My hosts were friendly and direct. They behaved naturally, in an open fashion, without superiority, disdain or condescension. I felt accepted at face value, without caveat. Nuances related to accent, class, rank or background were absent.

The abundance of supplies was striking following the scarcity to which we were accustomed. Everything American was in surplus. Personnel, transport, gasoline, liquor, tobacco, toilet rolls, soap, cash and a variety of delicious food constituted a quarter-master's paradise. By itself, this bounty would not win the war—killing the enemy was necessary for that—but it improved daily life.

My roommate was a native Californian and he described the Golden State from the Pacific shore to the high Sierras, from the redwoods and mountains of the north to the palm trees and deserts of the south. As I lay, listening and idly wondering whether to have another chocolate or a Virginia cigarette, a nascent thought arose: I must go to America.

My colleague, a lawyer, outranked me. (Among the U.S. plenty, lawyers were included, and as international collaboration was involved a lawyer was a logical choice.) He possessed diplomatic skills together with expertise in drafting documents. I knew the factors that governed bomb trajectories and could compose persiflage. Our synergy proved effective. At our first meeting we agreed on a conclusion, which we had formed singly: We did not believe any benefit would accrue by liaison on bombsights. On the contrary, we thought that attempts to forge any combination would be damaging. The mechanisms upon which the two instruments depended differed fundamentally. It was impossible to graft parts of one bombsight to the other. Pragmatic considerations weighed against an attempt. Mechanics were accustomed to the instruments and the aircraft had been modified to receive them. Air crew were trained to use them.

Dislocating this with the dubious prospect of a theoretical improvement would be foolish. (As the Americans say, "If it ain't broke, don't fix it.") But reaching this decision was only a fraction of our task. Parkinson's Law—which Mr. Parkinson devised, not surprisingly, as a result of his experience in the British War Office—was in operation: Work expanded to fill the time available. We made field trips, interviewing those who used, installed, and repaired bombsights. This brush with reality lent verisimilitude to our account, upon which we expended painstaking effort, particularly the summary, which we suspected would be the only section most people would read. We observed scrupulous balance between our respective Air Forces in reaching our wise conclusion: "Do nothing." We lavished care upon the stylish packaging of our report. I was promoted after we submitted our study, confirming the lyricist W. S. Gilbert's observation on the attributes necessary for advancement in the military. In fact, I had been the only beneficiary of this enterprise: My course was now set for America.

The military maxim: "Never volunteer" was familiar to me but I ignored it. The lure was London. A course was available there, and I volunteered despite a prediction from an experienced comrade that I would be transferred subsequently. He was correct. My orders read: "Report to RAF Katakurunda." I knew it was not in England and feared it was in Scotland or, worse, Ireland. Air Ministry informed me: "It is in Ceylon." I spent my embarkation leave at Wimbledon, where my brother introduced me to his girlfriend, Kate. She was fourteen to my twenty-one, tall, blonde, with a captivating smile.

England lay deep under snow as the aircraft, leaving at nightfall, carried me on the first leg of the long journey to the Far East. It was January 1945 and military aircraft were cold, noisy, uncomfortable and dangerous. We were a mixed bag of about a dozen, all male, on separate tasks, bound for different destinations. No details of itinerary had been provided and we were agreeably surprised when, following hours of flight all in darkness, we landed at dawn in Malta. The Mediterranean air was warm and soft, the people welcoming. Fresh fruit, cream and chocolates were served.

We left again at night, with a different contingent of passengers, our destination again unknown. We landed at Cairo, because one of the engines needed replacement, according to rumor, our only source of information. Scotch whisky at a nickel a shot is my only memory of the ancient city, as we were forbidden to leave the transit officers mess, the fiction being that the aircraft was liable to depart at a moment's notice. (As all combatants learned, waiting comprised the major part of war. Once, at a large gathering awaiting some commandant, the men sang, in unison, ponderously but with resonance to a hymnal tune I recognized, "Waiting, waiting, WAITING/Always bloody well waiting/Waiting in the morning/And at the close of day.") I played bridge profitably for several days and then was selected for the next eastbound aircraft. The priority system was a mystery to all. Rank played a part, but not the major one.

This flight began in the dark, the desert beneath us offering not a glimmer of light. We appeared suspended in the night, with only the comforting rhythm of the engines to reassure us. A man regaled me with tales of the fate awaiting anyone unfortunate enough to be captured by the dervishes should we make a forced landing. Rarely has sunrise been more welcome. As the thin gleams lit the desert I saw Baghdad.

We were a small party and shared a jitney with the air crew into the city, where we toured the bazaars. Several people purchased rugs, planning to sell them profitably in London, but I abstained. The weather was cool but sunny, but the dust, hubbub, press of humanity, together with music, jangling and discordant, were trying. This cacophony prevailed in all Oriental cities I visited.

When the plane door opened in Karachi the heat was fiery, no humidity but no shade, the baking sun reflected from the hard sand. I became lost in the town, the only white face amid brown; fierce, hawkish men striding past, women gliding quietly by, and hordes of children, laughing, playing, begging and dancing round me. We next reached Bombay, a romantic city. Marine Drive, which sweeps around the harbor, was cool, with a breeze off the ocean, welcome following the desert heat. I wore tropical kit and enjoyed the colors, spices and glamour of the city.

But this pleasure was short-lived, for I had fallen from grace with the air and was condemned to travel by troop train to Madras in southern India. An ancient locomotive spewing steam at every pore finally arrived at the Bombay station, and the troops were locked into third-class carriages, with wooden benches and little ventilation. Officers fared better, six to a compartment, but all shared the heat and delays as we steered south. The journey was punctuated by halts, some of minutes, several of hours, for no apparent reason. (Time in India was understood to be elastic, so haste was useless.) We made scheduled stops at railroad stations, and were allowed to leave the train. Railroad stations in India were large buildings in and around which many people of all ages lived, without any hope of travelling on a train or other conveyance.

The men were fed Army rations, and marched back and forth for exercise, but were not allowed to enter the station premises. The officers were permitted to buy food in the restaurants, which resembled those in London, except the latter were cold, drafty and quiet, whereas here it was hot, humid and noisy, yet the waiters spoke English. Never having seen, smelt, or eaten spicy food, I was new to curry. My companions advised me to take one bite of a banana per mouthful of curry to lessen its volcanic effect. The ventilation consisted of fans that often were stationary, as the electricity supply was fickle; the standby system was a drape that hung from the ceiling by pulleys. Two small boys walked the length of the room, one each side, to and fro, pulling this heavy contraption. The waiters scolded them, but the boys enjoyed a privileged position, being rewarded occasionally by tips and always with food.

The journey, or ordeal, lasted five days and nights, until we reached Madras. I had developed a skin rash and a sympathetic adjutant sent me to a transit camp near the ocean. The sea that girds the British Isles is cold in summer and frigid in winter: to paddle is ill-advised, to wade foolhardy, to swim insane. The Madras beaches were of soft white sand, sensuous to the feet. Rollers of blue water curled onto the beach. I swam in slow delight and floated, luxuriating in the warm Indian Ocean. Refreshed, I body-surfed, my energy restored. Following a few days in this Eden, my skin healed. I boarded a train which carried me further south to the port from which the ferry departed for Ceylon. I had reservations for a cabin on the ship and for a first class carriage on the train to Colombo, the capital. Then I learned that, mysteriously, the cabin was unavailable and the carriage nowhere to be found. Looking into the eyes of the ship's purser and the train's conductor, I read the same message. The sahib could pay to rectify the situation if he desired, or spend the night on the ship's deck.

This was my introduction to the manner in which business is conducted in the Orient, and I became versed in its nuances.

When I arrived at the RAF station, no one knew why I was there or what I was to do. This was solved by the onset of amoebic dysentery, for which I was treated in the Army hospital, a gracious old building with attractive gardens. There was only one other patient in the officers' ward, a captain in the Ceylonese Light Infantry who had a fever of unknown origin. He was from an old Ceylonese family, and a better companion I could not have found. Civilized, educated, refined, he was lonely and welcomed a companion, even one such as I, ignorant of his country and its history and culture. My treatment consisted of countless enemas so I was confined to bed for the first week. As I lay, he talked in his soft, sibilant voice, using precise English, describing the island. As I became stronger and able to walk and sit in the garden, I questioned him as he explained Buddhism, an ascetic mystical faith with an ethos that was pacifist, not warlike; the goal being to achieve nirvana, a state of mind reached by meditation. Contemplation of Buddhism must have been therapeutic, for we improved synchronously and were granted convalescent leave.

My new friend invited me to accompany him on a visit to the Highlands. Colombo was pleasant yet humid, but as we left the plains in his convertible and the road climbed amid the green hills the air became crisp and cool. We visited Kandy, a sacred city, where a religious procession was in progress. Elephants adorned by tapestries marched ponderously through the streets as the people threw flowers in their path and chanted amid the peal of bells and clash of cymbals.

We continued our journey, climbing to 6,000 feet among scenery that reminded me of the Scottish mountains. Pine trees were wreathed in cool mists that drifted down the valley. But unlike Scotland, the hillsides were covered with tea plantations. We reached Nuwara Eliya, the hill station where the English retreated to be out of Colombo in the hot season. We stayed at the Hill Club, a British oasis in this faraway scented isle. The furnishings, pictures, and the rituals of meals were copied from London, and the illusion of being in Pall Mall was sometimes complete; but then it would be shattered by a raucous cry from a tropical bird of a plumage never seen in St. James' Park, or dissolve in a glimpse of frangipani and orchids.

For the final week of convalescent leave we returned to Colombo, where I was billeted in the Galle Face Hotel. Occupying a superb site on a rocky promontory on the beach, it was a luxury establishment, with food and service to match. I joined two Australian officers to swim and enjoy the surf. Ignorant of the local waters, we were swept out to sea and I thought we would drown. A boat appeared, an outrigger with a single triangular sail, and two Ceylonese fisherman dragged us aboard, frightened, weak and waterlogged. In gratitude, we immediately promised them 500 rupees (150 dollars U.S.). They spoke little English but understood our pledge, altering course to deposit us at the hotel where our money was. As we neared shore and our strength and spirits rose, we decided we had been overly generous—why, we could have swum back, or drifted down the coast and escaped the rip tide and reached shore on our own. Nonetheless, we would pay our ransom, and with some difficulty were able to come up with 500 rupees between us. Our rescuers were outraged, insisting 500 rupees each had been promised. But at this blackmail, we stood our ground, for we were three to two, and white officers. They were brown and poor, and trespassing on the sahib's grounds. We prevailed.

When I finally reported for duty the adjutant had a job for me. My records, now received, revealed a degree in physics, so I was appointed education officer, with quarters in the library. In my new role I shared a difficulty with the chaplain, that of attracting an audience. So I catalogued the library, a pleasant task. In the mess I was classified with the medical officer and the chaplain, all over-educated. I also became a courier, flying to Delhi and Calcutta with documents not entrusted to the mail.

I had a manservant to whom I paid a pittance, the going rate, on which he supported his family. His dignity, care and devotion knew no bounds. My clothes were washed and ironed to perfection. He put toothpaste on my toothbrush, to spare me this chore. While I was undressing from uniform to pajamas he assisted. When putting on my trousers he knelt in front of me, asking me to put a hand alternately on each of his shoulders to steady myself while he pulled on each trouser leg. With his assistance one could make retiring a graceful act even when inebriated.

There was no enemy action in Ceylon. We mounted no bombing raids or fighter sorties. Coastal patrols and transport duties occupied the air crews. This idyll resulted in a sybaritic life, yet Eden was not perfect. Isolation, or island fever, affected us. Letters and newspapers were dated, radio news sparse. The war was approaching a climax in Europe and we were not part of it.

It was in Ceylon that I first experienced "entertainment for the troops." At the movies men made comments not ordinarily heard in the cinema. The conclusion of one film showed a sailing ship gliding into the sunset. From the shore the hero proclaimed, "Every man has one woman he loves and mine is on yonder ship." "And mine is in Leeds," yelled a soldier. Live shows were infrequent but entertainers did sometimes visit us. The setting was always the same—an outdoor stage, a tropical night and a packed audience. Seating was by rank: officers in front, then NCOs, the men at the rear, MPs strategically sited near the stage. While waiting, the troops sang their versions of "White Christmas" and other favorites.

One show featured a pair of dancers. The CO was particularly taken, bellowing and applauding conspicuously. At the conclusion of their act they disrobed on the stage, revealing balding scalps, hairy torsos and knobby knees. The CO was ill-tempered for days. The evening invariably ended with a sultry blonde singing "I'm in the mood for love." So was the audience.

In Burma, where I was later posted, one act created a sensation. Billed as a contortionist, a lithe dancer appeared, dressed in a flesh-colored transparent bodysuit. The lighting crew killed all but the two spotlights. The temperature of the audience rose, a testosterone miasma filled the air, silence was absolute. The woman began to dance, sinuously coiling and uncoiling her body—no bump and grind, but elegant movements, increasing in time with the piano tempo. The lights caressed her, colors changing with the mood. Finally the dance slowed and the piano ceased. The lights, white now, coned on her pelvis. Facing the audience, feet apart, she culminated with an agonizingly slow backward stretch, her palms on the floor behind her. A chord on the piano, house lights up and deafening applause. She conferred with her accompanist, then announced an encore. Amid the ensuing silence, a plaintive voice from the back called: "Please, miss, do it on the piano, I can't see."

I believe we were all grateful to the entertainers, who faced long, dangerous journeys, disease, and hardship, coupled with time away from their careers in an already precarious profession.

Some men who had been a long time overseas behaved oddly, perhaps as a coping mechanism. Some built walls, or peculiar edifices resembling temples, with beer cans or bottles. These structures were precious to them, and to denigrate them, or worse, damage them would have been foolhardy. Theft was endemic. I once shared a hut with an officer who would fire his pistol through the roof or walls at irregular intervals, as his mood dictated. It made for a disturbed night but no one ever stole anything from us.

In the Mess, to wear headgear at breakfast signified you did not desire conversation. Silence at breakfast is to be prized and I sometimes wish the custom had been adopted in civilian life.

Immediately following the Japanese surrender in August, 1945, I was posted to Penang and Malaysia for no apparent reason. Later I was sent to Singapore, whereupon landing at Changi airport we were not permitted to leave the arrival area for security reasons. Our landing immediately preceded that of Field Marshal Montgomery, who had had no hand in the Asian campaign. I observed him closely, being near enough to touch him. He was a small erect man with a cocky air, wearing tropical kit that revealed a tattoo on his forearm. Greeted by the General Officer Commanding Singapore, he paid him scant attention. An open staff car awaited the two men, pennants flying. Montgomery entered first. The G. O. C. attempted to follow, but found the door slammed in his face. Monty stood up alone in the car, waving to the soldiers, leaving his escorts stranded.

I suffered a recurrence of dysentery requiring hospitalization. Following recovery, my good fortune deserted me. I was sent to Burma, to an airfield between Rangoon and Mandalay. The terrain was inhospitable. The climate was vile: hot, humid, with torrential rains. We developed skin diseases and suffered from leeches. We lived in huts or under canvas. The food was poor and there was little recreation. The war was over, many were going home, but we were isolated and forgotten. The Burmese people were in dire straits and civil war appeared imminent.

— Antecedents —

I now received a communication from the King of England stating he could dispense with my services in the defense of the Realm, should I choose to be demobilized in Burma. I had had in mind separating from His Majesty's support in the vicinity of Piccadilly Circus, not Rangoon, and so elected to await shipping to the U.K.

I reverted to Armament Officer, responsible for a large cache of arms. As units were repatriated our airfield became the site of surplus ordnance and ammunition, some Japanese but the majority British. I then received a sensible order, to select sufficient arms for the protection of our personnel and airfield and to dispose of the surplus by air drop into the sea. We had few suitable aircraft but everyone worked hard, since it was clear that until this task was completed we would not be leaving.

Suddenly, an Air Commodore appeared and called for a description of the dumping operation. I had no experience of dealing directly with an officer of this rank. I described the procedure and proudly indicated our splendid progress. He demanded a detailed list of the weapons and ammunition already dropped, together with their identification numbers. I produced my order, pointing out that no mention was made of an itemized list or description.

This did not mollify him. Instead he became incensed. Dropping large quantities of His Majesty's property unrecorded into foreign waters was a court-martial offense, for which he would indict me when he reached London. He was a career officer facing reduction in rank now that the war was over. He sought some distinction to avert this and since it could no longer be obtained at the enemy's expense, it was to be at mine. No solution occurred to me except to add his body to the next consignment. In any event, he never acted on his threat. Two days later, deliverance came in the guise of the *S. S. Somersetshire* of the Bibby Line, which steamed up the river to our rescue. We, the RAF, were the first passengers, and thankfully boarded her, bound, at last, in the fall of 1947, for home.

The voyage was enjoyable at first. The tropical sea was calm, flying fish accompanied the ship, and our wake signified that each mile brought us nearer home. The nights were hot, so I slept on the deck, gazing at the starry floor of heaven where the Southern Cross shone brightly. But as we slowly steamed westward the ship made several stops, boarding many troops, and the Army assumed control.

Orderly officers' duties included the inspection of the prisoners, who were in small cells deep in the forecastle. They were returning to long incarceration in military jails. In response to the standard query: "Any complaints?" they always replied stoically, "No, Sir."

Light relief came when we entered the Suez Canal and a troupe of monkeys boarded the ship. The MPs' efforts to capture them were generally fruitless, for nature and the ship's superstructure gave the apes an overwhelming advantage. The men cheered and finally the MPs despaired of the unequal contest and left their ancestors alone. Rumor held that a bevy of ladies, under cover of this diversion, had also boarded and were plying their profession as we slowly traversed the canal, but sadly no further information was available, at least to officers. The ladies and apes disembarked at Suez, wisely deciding not to continue to Liverpool, our destination. In the Mediterranean the weather worsened, culminating in fierce storms in the Bay of Biscay. Our contingent had now been afloat for weeks and we had only tropical kit. As we slowly beat our way north, we were freezing.

We finally made landfall in Liverpool in November 1947. After three years' absence England seemed small, poor, grey, and cold. The demobilization staff were helpful and listed several jobs for which I might be suited, but I sought a new skill to enable me to prosper in the new country I had chosen. The British equivalent of the GI Bill offered that opportunity.

Chapter 3

Indoctrination

The Middlesex Hospital occupies a twenty-five-acre site near Soho, a raffish district in London. The hospital was founded in 1745, the Medical School ninety years later. The present building was completed in 1935, providing beds for 760 patients: a handsome structure in the form of a capital H, seven stories high. The size and profusion of the windows results in a generous spread of light. A courtyard garden is hidden within the center, with seats for the patients, staff, and students to enjoy the flowers and a soothing fountain. The library windows look out on this scene, which tends to distract those studying there. The outbuildings of the hospital are scattered throughout the tangle of streets around the main building, and include clinics, laboratories, classrooms, and, fortunately, a cafeteria.

The name "Middlesex" refers to the county of that name. (This is not clear to all. When two Americans walked by, one asked, "What's that place?" "The Middlesex Hospital," the other replied. "Gee, I didn't know there were enough of them to warrant a separate hospital," rejoined the first.)

The Medical School class of 1953 entered in June 1948 to start their five-year apprenticeship. The eighty students included eight women, the first to be admitted. Age divided the class into two parts—youngsters of nineteen newly graduated from high school, and an older group who had served in the war.

The curriculum decreed that we study anatomy and physiology for the first year, followed by pathology and pharmacology for the second. Our knowledge was then to be put to a stern test. A written and oral examination, administered by the University of London, would be posed to us and the students of seven lesser schools. It was essential to clear this hurdle in order to be admitted to the three clinical years, which would be spent walking the wards of the hospital.

The lectures and laboratory studies that confronted us caused me apprehension, with good reason. Four years in the RAF, where thinking was not encouraged, were unsuitable preparation for competing in unfamiliar subjects with students fresh from school. As time passed, the quantity of information imparted grew rapidly. Good health, stamina, equanimity and a sense of humor were essential, but these attributes alone might not prevail: I needed help.

Help came in the guise of Larry, my anatomy partner. (Our task was to dissect half of a cadaver and record the findings.) Larry had been in the Army, landed in Sicily and fought in Italy. He described the campaign for Monte Cassino, which provided light relief after hours of *Grey's Anatomy*. He finished in Germany with garrison duties, including a social life, which made for better telling than my stint in Burma. Larry was more intelligent than I, which was noted by several of our teachers; one, a Conan Doyle enthusiast, called him "Holmes" and me "Watson." Larry chose neurology, the intellectual specialty. Larry and I eventually extended our cooperation from anatomy to the whole curriculum, being together daily and working companionably in harness for five years, and I feel that without his friendship the outcome for me might have been different.

Anatomy posed a problem for me, for I cannot envision spatial relationships. (This disability is innate, as is, for example, color blindness.) The vessels, nerves, viscera, muscles, tendons, ligaments, ducts, integuments all coursed in a bewildering fashion that I could not fathom, retain, nor reproduce. My lack of drawing ability made this worse. The professor of anatomy, a Scot, was a key figure in our firmament. Each day was heralded by his lecture, lucid and illustrated by drawings in colored chalk on the blackboard. He never used slides or films. As the year progressed, I fell behind and resorted to coming into the dissecting room in the early evening and on Saturday morning. Our professor was often there, and once asked, "What are you doing?"

"Revising, sir," I replied.

"You cannot revise what you never vised," he responded tartly.

Anatomy demonstrated the structure of the body in health, physiology its functions. Our professor of physiology had a different style from our anatomy professor's. He used the Socratic method of question and answer, selecting puzzling or controversial points and illuminating them with provocative discussion. He was the author of the standard textbook and conscious of that distinction. After discussing the topic we would read the corresponding section of his book.

Physiology, in contrast to anatomy, deals with the dynamics of the body. It explores the self-regulating mechanisms that ensure internal stability, in response to normal stimuli. There is a coordinated reaction of the organs of the body to demands made on it. Cardiac and respiration rates fluctuate, together with blood pressure, in exercise and rest. Body temperature is controlled, as is the composition of body fluids within prescribed limits. Growth and cyclical changes are governed by the endocrine system. The nervous system orchestrates these changes without conscious effort on our part, waking or sleeping.

Among our class, a few personalities stood out. Belle, older than her peers, was married and rich. She made distracting noises—her elaborate dresses rustled, her high heels tapped, her jewelry tinkled. Her perfume was pervasive, emanating a distinctive musky aroma. (When trying to locate her I once asked the dour hall porter, "Mr. Brown, have you seen Belle?" "I ain't seen her, heard her, or smelt her," he replied.) She had style and a good line in repartee, which attracted our physiology professor. A typical exchange ran: "Please distinguish between adolescence and puberty?" "Certainly, sir. Adolescence is the time spent becoming accustomed to puberty."

In the hospital we were not only tolerated but treated as junior members of the Middlesex family. We participated in the social activities, integrated with students of the other schools. Nursing was the largest and most hardworking. Their shifts lasted twelve hours and they worked both days and nights in the hospital. They suffered lectures but the major part of their learning occurred on the wards under the watchful eyes of the ward sisters and staff nurses. The students lived in the nurses' home adjacent to the hospital and, to my knowledge, were seen only in uniform. Despite restrictions, they provided the ferment of the social events.

Parliament passed the National Health Service legislation, placing the hospital under political control. The first NHS administrator was not heralded with enthusiasm. He styled himself "Brigadier," perpetuating his Army rank. Some thought this pretentious, as had he been a corporal he would not have noted that on his letterhead. (Several of our teachers had held rank superior to his but none retained it and honors were common among our consultants but they carried them lightly. Two of the seniors were Lords and there were several Baronets, but when their titles were referred to, the holders were invariably self-deprecating in their response. It was not the custom to advertise your rank in the Middlesex galaxy.)

One Friday a gnome, garishly painted, was placed on the fountain pedestal in the courtyard garden. Rumor held that this unwelcome addition was erected on the Brigadier's orders, symbolic perhaps. We returned on Monday to find that the gnome had replicated itself. Copies appeared on prominent sites, particularly on high, inaccessible corners of the masonry. Their leader, taller than his followers, was on the capstone high over the entrance courtyard, and was conspicuous not only for his commanding position but also for his priapism. Strenuous efforts, presumably directed by the Brigadier, were made to dislodge the offenders; however, these efforts came to nothing because the hospital servants were loyal but not to the point of clambering along high ledges. Finally, the fire brigade came with their biggest ladder truck and pried the leading gnome from his perch amid loud jeers. The commotion drew a lunchtime crowd of spectators and, to the Brigadier's special chagrin, the press with photographers.

No one could explain how the gnomes were made or placed but some suggested they were made of orthopedic plaster. Among the students were some with rock-climbing experience who were reported to have scaled several prominent buildings in the older universities, in addition to natural obstacles. But official inquiries were fruitless. Cynics said the score was Students 1, Brigadier 0.

Recreation was needed as an antidote to study. At school I had played rugby football and learned to be a goal kicker, which attribute enabled me to keep a place in the hospital "FIRST XV" for five years. We faced many vaunted teams in London and England, but experience taught me to beware of lesser-known rivals for whom we were a prime target.

Wales, where rugby ranked with singing as sacrosanct, was the home of many such teams, manned by coal miners. The epitome was Maesteg, a small pit town in the heart of rugby country. We had to take a train before 6:00 AM for the five-hour journey, and, when we arrived it was raining, as is usual there. Our hosts took us for a walk around town, built on a hill, in order to stretch our legs. We did not eat before a game and, having risen before the sun, were tired, hungry, and wet on arrival at the field. The visitors' changing room was in the basement of the wooden stand, which was packed with their supporters. While waiting they sang in Welsh and stamped their feet in unison.

One season, wishing to reassure our new young quarterback, I visited him while we were changing. Shouting some platitude above the singing and stamping did not console him—he replied, "Only the laundry knows how scared I am."

When we reached the pitch there were two minutes of silence in respect for some worthy supporter who had died. This ensured that our backs, on whose speed and handling we relied, were numb with cold and soaking wet.

Maesteg's forwards, I became convinced, had been kept down in the coal mine all week only to be released on Saturday to demolish us. They were short, swarthy men, unshaven, with a coarse black stubble on their rock-like chins. During the scrums they rubbed these needles up and down against our faces like a beast scouring itself on a tree trunk. Already possessing a cauliflower ear and broken nose, I still resented this attack on my features. They muttered curses in Welsh interspersed with English. I would have played three hours against any of the English clubs rather than an hour and a half versus Maesteg.

After the game all was bonhommie. A fry-up was followed by beer accompanied by stories and songs. We were sad to leave. They guided us to the station and waved farewell to the stopping train, which deposited us, sore and exhausted, at five on Sunday morning in London. Skeptics might say, "Lost to Maesteg! Whoever heard of Maesteg?" Little did they know.

Our dog, a retriever sometimes answering to the name of Mugs, needed walking, which duty fell to me. We met a black spaniel and the two dogs acted like old friends. The spaniel's owner, Kate Macnamara, appeared, a tall blonde with a brilliant smile, tantalizingly familiar. We had met, it transpired, four years previously for tea at our house when she was my brother's guest. He was now at college in Switzerland and had carelessly left his possessions unattended. It was my duty to act as her companion during his absence.

We exchanged news. She was seventeen, in her last year at school, and yearned to become a doctor, but the obstacles to entering medical school appeared insurmountable as only one place in ten was reserved for women. The first task was to place high in the examination in order to be in contention. However, as all those considered had done the same, something extra was needed in order to be singled out.

One fact was clear. The Dean alone determined who was to be admitted, and that decision was based on interviews. But, as he could not interview all applicants, some preliminary screening had to be done. The Dean's secretary controlled access to both the people and the papers that reached him, so I presumed that she selected applications, which were placed on his desk. Our problem was simplified—it was necessary to influence these two individuals with subtlety.

I had not met the secretary, for I had encountered no difficulties requiring her attention, which was fortunate. I requested an interview and, disingenuously, presented my petition. A young lady, a friend of mine, no, a friend of the family really, had applied for admission as I had told her the Middlesex was the best school in London, indeed in England. So I felt responsible in a way and wanted to ensure that her documents were in order. I thought I detected a twinkle in the secretary's eye as she asked the name. She warned me that, of course, all contenders were treated equally, but said she would read her application.

The Dean was a baronet and a rugby fan who attended games. He did not sit sensibly in the stand with his peers, but patrolled the touch line, shouting advice, fielding the ball, throwing it back, sometimes trying a kick and getting muddy. He joined us at tea following the game. What more natural than that Kate should come to our games, applauding from the touchline and serving tea?

Kate described her interview. The Dean, trained in observation as all good doctors are, looked closely at her as she smiled at him. "Haven't we met before?"

"Yes, sir."

"Don't tell me, wait." His clinical acumen did not fail him. "At the rugby matches."

"Yes, sir."

"You like rugby?"
"Yes, sir."
"And support our team?"
"Yes, sir."
"Thank you, good day."

Twenty-seven years later Kate served on the admissions committee of the Johns Hopkins University School of Medicine, together with twenty fellow faculty members. Assisted by staff, including a lawyer, they toiled long and hard to identify those applicants most deserving of admission and to reject those of lesser merit. Scholarly papers, none of which mention cost, demonstrate that this method is nearest to perfection in this imperfect world. Maybe so, but as for me, I bet on the Dean. We kept in touch with his secretary long into her retirement, sending pictures of our growing family and news of our checkered careers, for both of which her intuition and intervention had been in part responsible.

In our second year we studied pharmacology. This entailed grasping certain principles, together with a mass of detailed information, much of which was imparted by lecture. We were singularly fortunate in our teacher, a doctor who understood that in order to instruct one must first entertain. Our lecture room, on an upper floor of the hospital, had open windows in the hope that ventilation would keep us awake. One day, in the midst of a difficult topic, we heard a loud crash of broken glass from the courtyard below. "Don't worry, merely a dissatisfied patient disposing of a bottle of medicine," was the professor's explanation.

Between the pages of his lectures our teacher slipped vivid examples of how doctors should conduct themselves. He had once held the post of casualty medical officer, the first person to see emergencies. He sometimes made house calls in the vicinity. One morning, answering the telephone, he heard a voice begin, "The Duke of Bedford—."

"Right away," interrupted our hero, hanging up on the caller, grabbing his medical bag, and darting out the door on the way to the pub of that name. (Our hospital was surrounded by pubs in alleys, courts, squares, and byways.) But the pub he arrived at proved to be the Duke of York, not of Bedford. Not wishing to appear rude by immediately inquiring about the location of a rival establishment, he ordered a pint and gulped it down.

"Duke of Bedford," pondered the landlord. "I'm not quite sure, but it can't be far. Go to the Queen's Head across the square. The landlord was born near here, he'll know." Arriving there, our teacher prudently had half a pint, then inquired. The landlord being out, the barmaid was anxious to help and canvassed the regulars, who eventually reached a consensus. They insisted he have the other half pint while they imparted a series of complicated directions. Leaving the Queen's Head, he was soon lost and took refuge in the King's Arms. Being full of beer but low in spirits, he had a large whisky, then made his inquiry. "The Duke of Bedford is three miles from here," stated a man, with conviction.

Disconsolate, our professor meandered back to the hospital, to be met by his irate chief, who announced, "While you've been out getting drunk, the Duke of Bedford has died in your casualty ward."

Our teacher also impressed on us the need to consider the viewpoint of patients. For example, if a man states that he has a headache, that is a fact. If you can find no organic cause for it, that can be reassuring if explained to the patient clearly, but it does not mean he does not have a headache. It simply means you cannot uncover the reason for it. You talk to the patient in that light, discuss it with him, and he tells you the cause of the headache.

When making rounds we were told to sit down at the patient's bedside. This gives people the impression that you have time for them, which is not conveyed by remaining standing. When talking with the patient, provide an area of psychological privacy, such as two chairs in a corner. You should concentrate on the patient, listen to her, look into her eyes as if you two were the only people in the world. "Always touch the patient," he advised, "hold their hand, press it in both of yours."

Our teacher warned us about the braggart who says—"Doc, nothing is too good for Grandma—only the best, you understand." This means you won't be paid, nor will the hospital, and the relatives will never take Grandma back. In contrast, the anxious relatives who say, "We don't know how we will pay for this or look after her," mean they'll do both, as only the good worry.

Our professor never put his patients on a diet, declaring it only made them anxious and eat more. He was the only teacher who talked to us about death. The job of certifying the death of a patient in hospital falls to the junior doctor. We were cautioned to take our time, especially in the geriatric ward, as vital signs in the very old are irregular and can deceive the unwary. If you have any doubt, wait. If you declare the patient to be dead and start the paperwork, your reputation is also dead should the patient suddenly wake and ask for a cup of tea. But if the patient is dead your duty is over.

Never attend patients' funerals. Early in his career he had not followed this precept. Receiving a garbled message that a patient was in imminent danger of death, he made a prompt house call. The address was in Covent Garden market and proved to be a six-story walkup. Arriving breathless in a small room, he found a corpse, dead for some hours as evidenced by rigor mortis. Also present were two drunken men. Our doctor said: "This man is dead, there is nothing I can do," and made to leave.

"'Ere, 'ere, not so fast, you've come too late, you 'ave, and now you say you can't do nothing," Fred, the larger of the two, exclaimed.

"We're the only friends he's got," added the smaller man, starting to cry.

"You should have acted sooner," responded the doctor.

"We tried to, we knew he was sick. Fred went out, couldn't find nobody who'd help, so he brought back a bottle or two so we could think what to do."

"Well, now you're 'ere at last, the least you can do is give us a hand," said Fred. Whatever had killed their friend, it was not malnutrition, for he weighed about 250 pounds. Our teacher now found himself one of a trio carrying the corpse down the six flights. It was no easy task. The narrow staircase twisted, the corpse was huge and rigid, and two out of the three pallbearers were drunk and distraught.

Gratefully reaching the street, the doctor said, "I'll call an ambulance."

"No you won't," retorted Fred. "We got here all right. Undertaker's just round the corner."

"We're the only friends he's got," reiterated Bill. "We'll have to pay for his funeral." They had cash and carry in mind, a cut rate. It was busy in the market and spectators crowded round, quickly realizing they were not witnessing a miracle of medical science.

Before the war, graduating classes had endured a commencement speech, sometimes lasting half an hour, but our teacher's effort won the prize for brevity. He said: "Congratulations, gentlemen, you are now empowered to sign death certificates. Please do so—sparingly. Good day."

Pathology, the study of the origin and nature of disease and its effects on the body, was our major subject during the second year. The Middlesex had just decided to send some students to affiliated hospitals in London and elsewhere for parts of their clinical work. Pathology was included and an opportunity to study at the Central Middlesex Hospital was open for two students. Larry and I were selected.

In this hospital, situated in a poor suburb of London, the patients, their diseases, and their doctors differed from those at the Middlesex. The patients were all poor, providing us our first insight into the effect of poverty upon health. They had common diseases, whereas many of those at the Middlesex had rare conditions, puzzling to diagnose and difficult to treat. The doctors at the Middlesex had practices in Harley Street, an address signifying that they had reached the pinnacle of success, in addition to their teaching duties. Those who now taught us worked only at the hospital, and saw disease as just one of the many burdens their patients bore.

Directly we reported to our teacher, the Chairman of Pathology, it was clear we were fortunate. Dr. Walter Pagel loved pathology. A small, intense man, he spoke with a guttural German accent despite having lived many years in London. Born and trained in Germany, the birthplace of pathology, he was full of infectious enthusiasm.

Greeting us warmly, he said to me, "You are the bearer of a famous name. Richard Morton wrote a thesis on phthisis" [using the original term for tuberculosis]. Diving into a pile of old books, he produced a dusty tome, and, sneezing triumphantly, turned to the pages written by my namesake.

He did not mention hours of attendance, duties, curriculum, textbooks, lectures or examinations, but immersed us immediately in the study of pathology. His responsibilities were many, including the laboratories where all the tests on blood, fluids, and tissue were performed and surgical specimens examined. He supervised the work done there, but his real love was the autopsy rooms adjacent to the hospital mortuary, situated in a discreet corner of the large grounds.

The hospital, a Victorian structure resembling a penitentiary, housed over a thousand beds. Most of the patients were old, and many were terminally ill as it was the hospital of last resort for the area it served. Autopsies were performed every morning, several in progress simultaneously. The junior pathologists performing these were supplied with the medical history of the patient and records of the last admission. We sifted the notes for relevant information or put on gloves to slice the lungs or the liver, searching for nodules if the doctor had suspected them in either organ during life. This taught us gross pathology in a realistic, firsthand way.

Dr. Pagel arrived in mid-morning, circulated, and selected interesting findings that he could discuss at the conference, which began at noon. The doctors who had cared for the patients attended and gave a brief history and their opinion as to the cause of death. The key organs were kept covered, so elements of detection and suspense were introduced. The pathologist, the doctors' doctor, had the last word, with the benefit of hindsight. Dr. Pagel presided, always sympathetic to the clinician, sometimes displaying his erudition, often remaining silent while his juniors summarized.

The surgical deaths were the highlight of the morning. Physicians are tolerant of death, surgeons are not, as they regard it as a defeat and a slight to their reputations. They had to make a preoperative diagnosis, which, in 1949, included some skillful guessing. If the post-operative findings did not confirm their pre-operative opinion, they were defensive, if not disbelieving. As the patient was dead, all agreed on that, it was difficult to present the case as a surgical triumph.

The operative site was always dissected and examined, for the surgeon was interested in this above all else. In the majority of cases the operation had been successful, but the patient died of medical complications. Dr. Pagel discussed the cases of the senior surgeons, his peers. Their exchanges were models of diplomatic comportment.

We enjoyed a late brown bag lunch with our mentor following the conference, sitting companionably in his office. He talked of the morning cases or, rarely, his other passion, opera. I prudently stayed silent, but Larry kept his end up. He had served in Salzburg and spoke a little German, which Pagel enjoyed. The afternoon was devoted to histology, the microscopic examination of the cells of an organ, which were stained with dyes better to delineate the details. The images, in varying degrees of magnification, were projected onto a screen in a darkened room while Dr. Pagel dictated a description and his diagnosis. The history of each patient was supplied and it was our duty to study this, give a synopsis, and be ready to answer any queries. Our teacher used a pointer to identify which cells he was describing. Kidney, brain, bone, liver, heart—all the organs of the body passed our review. As we improved, he taught us to identify pathological changes in cells—cancer first, as it is distinctive, followed with other, subtler processes.

The mortuary attendant was a former sergeant major, not in the Army but in the Guards. When the autopsies were finished, we helped him clear up, rather a morbid task. He was hospitable and repaid us in beer, which was welcome, but the utensils he served it in were questionable to say the least. They had contained specimens, of that we were certain; how well they had been cleaned we were not. As it is unwise to differ with a guards sergeant, especially one who is in charge of your work place, we downed the beer and our suspicions. We sometimes played tennis on the adjacent court. He would stand in the mortuary doorway, watching, and shout, as only a sergeant major can, "Any two in here could beat you."

The causal link between cigarette smoking and lung cancer was to be forged simultaneously in London and New York. Our hospital was the pathological center for the London investigation, and one of the large wards, containing forty beds, was set aside for this. As death approached, the patients were moved to the head of the ward adjacent to the corridor and nursing station. Our job was to elicit smoking histories from them. We crouched over them, straining to hear their answers to our questions. All were short of breath and they panted, struggling to inhale sufficient air to speak. Their replies were interrupted by bouts of blood-stained coughing, and some had had laryngectomies and had to scribble their answers.

We joined the rounds made by the cardiologist, Dr. Horace Joules, a good teacher. He was a big man, six feet six inches tall, with an avuncular, reassuring manner. He certainly touched his patients, placing his large hand squarely on their heads. Patients frequently asked: "What's wrong, Doctor, is it my heart?"

"Well, your heart is as old as you are," he would boom in response.

He taught us that recognition is the basis of diagnosis. You recognize a disease as you recognize a friend, a building, a painting, or the barking of your dog. He demonstrated it slowly for us, assembling each piece. The history, risk factors, signs, symptoms, course of the disease, test results, all taken together enable you to identify the disease.

It reminded me of the way we learned to recognize enemy aircraft during the war. First they showed us pictures of these aircraft, taken from many angles, when they were motionless. Then they showed us silhouettes, together with posted specifications, dimensions, equipment, armament, speed, range, and altitude limits. This was followed by a film showing the aircraft in flight, straight and level, in a sunny, cloudless sky. But at the same time we all knew that in combat, it is vital to recognize an aircraft instantly by one distinctive feature; a tailfin, engine nacelle as it dives out of a cloud above, below, or behind you. And so it is in medicine. Not every symptom and sign accompanies every case of the disease. You recognize the whole, in whatever guise it may appear, by one or two characteristic parts.

Dr. Joules taught me a second important concept. All his patients had heart disease; the majority were in heart failure due to a few common causes. Owing to his stimulus, I read a textbook that described rare conditions in addition to the common ones we saw. When called upon to give the diagnosis in a patient whom I had examined, I chose a rare condition that I had never encountered but which, to my inexperienced eye, appeared to fit.

Our teacher, not humbling me in front of my peers, drew me aside and we walked to the window overlooking the hospital gardens. Gazing out, he asked, "Can you see an eagle?"
"No, sir."
"What do you see?"
"Sparrows, sir."
"What is the diagnosis?"
"Congestive cardiac failure, sir. Due to mitral stenosis."
"Yes. Common things commonly occur."

This dramatic illustration of the statistical concept of probability and its role in differential diagnosis stayed with me. Fifteen years later, in 1965, I was the only obstetrician in a small town in the Pacific Northwest.

— Indoctrination —

Success is remembered, failure forgotten, so I can recall the only correct medical diagnosis I ever made where others failed.

Some diseases are protean. They manifest in varying forms according to which body system is affected. Historical examples include syphilis and tuberculosis, and AIDS today, all present in many guises, concealing their identity.

One of my patients brought her daughter to consult me. The history was pertinent and involved. Puberty was normal and menstruation regular at first. She attended college at UCLA, where she met her husband, a microbiologist. Shortly after their marriage she accompanied him on field trials in South America, her first experience overseas, where they lived in villages and worked in the bush. They had practiced barrier contraception but discontinued this on leaving the U.S. She had become ill, with weight loss and occasional temperature elevation. Her periods were irregular and scanty, then ceased. She had a fast pulse, attributed to an underlying unspecified infection. Her husband wanted her to return to the U.S. for diagnosis and treatment but she resisted this, wanting to stay with him and not disrupt his work. She became anxious over this early discord in their marriage and felt a failure, but pointed out that, despite her illness, she remained energetic. She was referred to tropical disease experts in South America on the assumption that they would be familiar with infections that might afflict newcomers who lived in remote rural areas. A pregnancy test was negative and many other diagnostic tests were performed, all directed toward identifying the infection that presumably accounted for her weight loss, fast heart rate, and occasional rise in temperature. The results were equivocal. Treatment with antibiotics was tried, to no avail.

They then returned to UCLA, where there are tropical medicine specialists. These doctors reviewed the medical dossier she had accumulated, repeated some tests and introduced new ones. They did not reach a consensus. She became more anxious and resorted to a visit to Mother. I heard all this with a sinking heart, for I knew little or nothing of tropical disease, so how could I succeed where the elite had failed? I skimmed through the daunting records, confused by the tests and titers, unfamiliar to me. I knew a physical exam, particularly pelvic, would reveal little of value, but I wanted to talk to her alone, without her mother, who had been augmenting her story. I asked Mother to excuse us while I performed the examination.

When we were alone I asked if there was anything else she could tell me, anything she might have overlooked or possibly withheld while her mother was present. I was watching her closely as she replied, thoughtfully, "No, I don't think it's Mom that makes me so jittery."

Suddenly I knew she was a sparrow, not an eagle. Recognition: there was one cardinal symptom that fitted, all the rest was camouflage.

I examined her, my heart beating as fast as hers. I ordered a blood test and asked them to return shortly, saying that I suspected she had a common condition that could be treated successfully.

Thyrotoxicosis presents in different ways and patients frequently suffer a long time before some complication leads to the correct diagnosis. President Bush was a case in point, a man under constant scrutiny, exhibiting for all to see the hyperactivity that accompanies the disease. Yet only when he suffered a cardiac complication did the investigation of the heart condition lead to the diagnosis of the underlying thyrotoxicosis.

In October 1949 Kate was admitted to the Medical School. She was delighted to exchange school uniform for the relaxed dress of a medical student and to set foot early on the road to emancipation.

We lived two blocks apart. I had been commuting on the subway, which entailed a tiring journey during which it was difficult to study. Spurred by the prospect of a traveling companion, I bought, for thirty pounds (fifty dollars), a 1936 Morris 8 convertible. The 8 referred not to the number of cylinders, but, optimistically, to the horsepower. The car had several virtues, being small, nimble, and beat up—ideal for the city. It could not go fast enough to get a ticket and was easy to push. If it should "fail to proceed," as Rolls Royce said about their cars, I had a tow rope stowed away. The car seated two, in intimacy with the hood up and in style with it down, British racing green showing its lines to advantage.

The courtyard in front of the hospital was for consultants' parking only. Their Rolls, Bentleys, Daimlers, and Lagondas glistened. Mac, a sergeant from the Irish Guards, genially presided, with his medals shining and his cockaded hat ready to doff to his clients. I waited until early evening, when he had just returned from the hospital pub, the One Tun, following his first pint.

"Mac, permit me to introduce a new student, Miss Macnamara."
"Welcome me darling, you're a lovely colleen."
"And this is our new car."
"In the emerald green, so it is."
"Wouldn't have it otherwise."

Upon this happy note we reached an Irish agreement. "Although it is strictly forbidden, you understand," explained Mac, "you could park provided you arrived before eight and left after six." He put the car in a corner. This amicable arrangement lasted four years, reaffirmed with Guinness, Gaelic songs, and gifts to mark St. Pat's and Christmas.

The morning journey provided me a valuable revision in first-year subjects. As she discussed her studies, Kate taught and questioned me. I also benefited by observing and trying to emulate her study habits, which were systematic and effective, in contrast to mine. We stayed late, studying in the library, and then, after the traffic had dispersed, enjoyed the trip home. Sharing the driving and use of the car was efficient and relaxing. I gave Kate advice on how to cope in the first year, which topics should not be missed and which might be.

Some evenings Kate was mysteriously occupied and, inexplicably, away for weekends, missing rugby games. I could understand that, at eighteen, the monopoly of her scarce leisure time by one male was boring and that experimentation was to be expected. But understanding was one thing, acceptance quite another. My concentration was disturbed. In study, this was of little consequence; however, on the rugby field it mattered, as I missed an easy kick and then a second. This fallibility was noticed, the diagnosis made, and corrective action taken. The suitors were identified, a resident doctor and two students. David, our larger tackle, had a word with each of them in the privacy of the men's room, and Kate's studies were no longer distracted by outside influences.

The burden of the increasing quantity of information that she had to assimilate was decisive. As medicine tightened its grip and ambition grew, she had no time nor energy to spare for new suitors. Propinquity was paramount in her choice of life's companion, lust in mine.

During the final scene of the last act of "My Fair Lady," Professor Higgins eventually realized his predicament and declaimed, "Damn, damn, damn, damn." I was not as tardy, summoning up my courage in

May 1952 to propose—marriage, I hasten to add. The fountain in the hospital courtyard garden provided the setting.

At the end of our second year I sat the examination. It was vital to pass, for I knew if I did not, my career in medicine was over. I felt confident in physiology, pharmacology, and pathology but dreaded anatomy. Again, I haunted the dissection room. "What is worrying you?" inquired the professor.

"The exam, sir."

"I dislike examinations," he replied, "but I distrust those who cannot pass them."

I did poorly on the six-hour written test and all hinged on the oral, which was held on a Monday morning following a weekend racked by worry. We were to be examined in our laboratory, which contained dissected cadavers, specimens of organs, and microscopic slides for identification. There were to be two examiners—an anatomist from another university, and our professor.

My oral began with only me and the visiting anatomist in the room. The stranger was a small, delicate man and I loomed over and around him. He diagnosed me in one glance—"brawn, beer, and no brains"—and selected the foot for the test. My spirits fell further, for it had never been my favorite structure. Stumbling and mumbling my way along, I felt all was lost.

Then our professor arrived and greeted me: "Mr. Morton, you look wan."

"Yes, sir."

"Did we not beat Guy's Hospital on Saturday?"

"Yes, sir."

"Did you not kick a goal or two?"

"Yes, sir."

"Well, it's always good to beat Guy's." He looked me straight in the eye and, figuratively, put his arm around me. "Now, upon what have you been enlightening our visitor?"

"The foot, sir."

"Ah! fascinating, but not your first love I fancy."

"No, sir."

He walked among the exhibits, pausing momentarily beside the skull with open cranium, said, "Ah no," and stopped between two pelvises, male and female. "Let us study the female pelvis. I suspect you have gained at least a social contact with some of its contents."

Such a risqué comment, out of character, astonished me. I had already decided which specialty to follow. He indicated the structures, in logical sequence, for me to identify. As I intoned the familiar litany—uterus, Fallopian tube, ovary, broad, round and uterosacral ligaments—and described their vascular and nerve supply, my confidence slowly returned.

He resumed: "Why is it thus?"

"For procreation," I answered.

We moved to embryology and difficult questions were asked, some of which he answered himself as he explained the errors that occur in development and lead to congenital defects of the newborn. Finally, we shared a microscope and I identified and described the cells, differentiated, each with a unique function to perform. We viewed primordial cells of the ovary, hidden and waiting for their growth and the moment when new life will be created. We saw cells of the Fallopian tube, capable of delicate movement that transfers the fertilized ovum down to the safety of the uterus, where the lining is prepared every month for the nurture of the embryo. We studied the cells of the cervix, arranged in armored layers, guarding the entrance to the genital tract. After we had shared these mysteries my professor departed, saying, "Well, you survived that ordeal."

The professor became the next Dean. Never was an appointment so richly deserved. Twelve years later, on my first return to England, we met. I opened the conversation with some trite remark on the changes in London. "Aye," he replied, "I cannot tell the lads from the lassies and I am an anatomist."

I took my medicine in one gulp, choosing a six-month clerkship under the senior physician. He was the last of the generalists; his peers were specializing in cardiology, neurology, endocrinology, and the like. He was a small, upright figure, distinguished by a disproportionately large skull. His manners were of an earlier era, his diction clear, conveying his opinion with detail and precision. His medical knowledge was encyclopedic and his textbook of medicine, of which he was the sole author, displayed it. He had also written a companion work, *Applied Medicine*, which comprised a series of case presentations, each telling a story with sufficient facts and clues provided to enable the reader to reach the right diagnosis or to answer correctly the questions he posed. This book provided a novel, entertaining, and effective method of teaching, the only example of its kind I encountered. Years later, when writing a textbook, I tried to emulate, both on paper and on computer, his interactive approach.

The professor arrived precisely at ten each morning, stepping down from his old Rolls, to be met by his intern, who took his hat, cane, and attaché case. His apparel never varied, a dark suit with a carnation in the lapel. The Head Porter would meet him in the hall and conduct him to the elevators in the medical wing, which were large. The porter would commandeer one, evict any occupants, and the doctor, accompanied by his intern, would enter. The porter operated the elevator and the trio rode, nonstop, to the top floor. Silence prevailed during this ritual. On reaching the ward, he was greeted by his Ward Sister, his retinue assembled, and rounds began. Lesser mortals called this spectacle ridiculous but I suspect it had a purpose. He was about to perform and needed to rid his mind of details and concentrate, to prepare to analyze and communicate. In later years I copied his method, not his ritual, by observing a moment or two of complete concentration before starting a lecture.

His patients varied in age, sex, and background, the majority referred by other doctors, and some coming from overseas specifically to consult him. They all shared puzzling histories and confusing symptoms where several diagnoses had been made and rejected, and treatments started, then altered and discarded. Tropical diseases were not uncommon. Patients were assigned to students and we were the first to interview and examine them, recording our findings in a prescribed manner. On rounds, the new patients were discussed first and we recited the history, physical findings, and test results. This was an ordeal but it taught me how to present a case systematically. He usually listened in silence but would occasionally interject a question, the nature of which was sometimes surprising, appearing unrelated to the case. "How old is her cat?" "When did he return from Africa?" "For how long has she been an alcoholic?" "When did this patient last attempt suicide?" His questions reminded me of observations made by Sherlock Holmes on meeting his clients in Baker Street.

His reputation attracted post-graduate students from the old British Empire. They came to London to sit the MRCP (Member of the Royal College of Physicians) exam, an essential qualification to become a consultant, and prized overseas for its immutable quality. Indians, Australians, Egyptians, and others joined rounds during the pre-exam session. One such occasion was the only instance in which the professor displayed emotion. The diagnosis was clear, megaloblastic (pernicious) anemia. This condition had been treated since 1926 with liver extract, a tedious and distasteful therapy. Our chief selected a young Australian doctor, bursting with health and energy, beaming from the front row.

"Doctor, how pray would you treat this patient?" he inquired. "I would be modern, sir, and use vitamin B12," came his confident answer. Although this was correct, it was clear immediately that one unnecessary word had been used. Two red blotches appeared on the professor's face as he made a conscious effort to compose himself.

"We are fortunate today to be enlightened by one from the antipodes," he opened. "Tell us, please, from which tissues B12 was isolated, when, and where reported?"

His victim could not call this to mind, and was told it was from kidney and liver in 1948 and reported in *Science*. "As you advise using modern therapy, please name the metallic ion on which the molecule is based?"

Silence from the antipodes.

"Cobalt," he answered his own question. This unequal contest drew to a timely end, and the Australian probably wished himself back on Bondi Beach or even Ayers Rock.

Our teacher was a biochemist, a distinction held by few at that time. He did not advertise this accomplishment, revealing it only as he explained biochemical pathways and associated cellular changes. Although biochemistry is one of the two pillars of modern medicine, the second being genetics, we received no formal teaching in either subject. Our teacher was far ahead of his day, but this was not evident by first impressions.

Rounds finished at noon and during the afternoons we attended the medical outpatient clinics, conducted by senior registrars, who are one rank below consultants. Here we saw a wide spectrum of patients, the majority with common diseases. The vicissitudes of city life resulted in overrepresentation of stress-related conditions and illnesses from excessive cigarette smoking and alcohol use. These six months were the closest I came to experiencing general medical practice.

Dances were held on most Saturdays in the cafeteria. The hospital hosted an annual Ball organized by the students, held in the Dorchester or Grosvenor Hotels. The tariff for the consultants and other luminaries was high but student tickets were not. The organizers retained some spares, which they sent to our seven sister schools, and this largesse resulted in our receiving invitations to their Balls. In five years my tuxedo saw much service.

The Middlesex promoted an annual variety show held at the Scala Theater, our neighbor. The proceeds were donated to the Cancer Society and the artists gave their services. The event attracted a glamorous audience. The consultants supported it generously and the medical students organized it. This arrangement was agreeable to both parties, the affluent and the impecunious. We greeted the guests, valet-parked the cars of those lacking chauffeurs. We were ushers, the nurses were program sellers, and both staffed the bars. Best of all, we ran the party in the Green Room following the performance. There, the histrionic and medical talent mingled, to round off an enjoyable evening.

At Christmas, the nursing and medical students gave a concert featuring skits lampooning our teachers. During one of the scene changes a trio of comely nurses emerged, dressed in scrub suits, fresh from the operating room. "God, what a mess," exclaimed the first, slowly drawing a cigarette pack from her stocking top as the second pulled a lighter from her bodice. When all three were smoking, exhaling slowly, a spotlight illuminated the new surgeon, seated with his wife in the third row.

First nurse: "Have you seen the new young surgeon?"
Second nurse: "Yes, he dresses so well."
Third nurse: "And so quickly."

Christmas at the hospital retained much of its magic, with none of the commercialism that now dominates it. The holiday was heralded by each ward giving a party, all held on the same evening. The prescribed route for guests in order to finish the course was to start on the top floor of the medical wing of the hospital and wend their way down. The parties given by the physicians were elegant, marked by witty conversation and medical jokes. As much attention was given to nutrition as hydration.

Consequently, six stops could be negotiated with dignity and one arrived on the ground floor safely, in good fettle for the ensuing test. This comprised crossing over to the surgical wing and climbing up six floors with a stop at each ward, thus avoiding offending anyone. Elegance was not much in evidence, particularly as the parties were now in full swing. If there was anything edible it had disappeared, but Christmas cheer was abundant. Reaching the operating rooms on the seventh floor constituted a stress test, survival of the fittest, which was just as well, for the anesthesiologists were hosts who viewed consciousness in their guests as a challenge. The potions they offered were to be taken sparingly.

The wards were decorated, especially the children's. The nurses provided a joyous spectacle on Christmas Eve, wearing their red cloaks, carrying lighted candles, and moving in procession through the wards, carolling. On Christmas Day a feast was served, the turkey carved by the senior physician in each ward. The patients were served by the nursing and medical students, who disposed of any remains. The patients who were able, on foot or in wheelchairs, visited the other wards, and good will prevailed.

Surgery fascinated me—action and drama in a small theater where I could play a minor part. I started with a month in neurosurgery, where the professor was reputed to be eccentric. His specialty was intracranial tumors. The patient was placed in a chair and the brain exposed. The professor and his assistant worked delicately, dissecting sections of the brain, while my task was to hold retractors and use the sucker to keep the operating field dry. The theater was almost in darkness, the overhead floods were never used. The three of us and the scrub nurse wore small lights on head bands, which projected a thin, intense beam directly on the area under dissection. This created a weird scene, accentuated by classical music playing in the background. I enjoyed the setting and it was the first time I had the opportunity to listen to good music at length.

The procedures were prolonged, frequently lasting eight hours. Surgery started early and I left home at 6:00 AM, causing me to miss my customary substantial breakfast. By lunchtime I was starving and worrying that this condition was audible to my co-workers. One day in the middle of an operation the professor suddenly announced that today was the

— INDOCTRINATION —

anniversary of the birth of the father of neurosurgery, Harvey Cushing of Johns Hopkins Hospital in Baltimore. To celebrate we would share a bottle of wine, a special vintage, as we worked.
"Just the ticket, in the nick of time," I thought. "Good old Harvey." All I could recall from our nutrition lectures was that alcohol was a ready source of calories and that it lacked fat and cholesterol, which sounded to me like an ideal food.

The circulating nurses opened a large bottle, the professor proposed a toast, we echoed it, and he took the first drink from a straw. Then it was passed to the nurses, the anesthesiologist, and the surgical assistant, all of whom took brief sips. At last the bottle reached me. As we were masked, I turned away, my back to the surgeon, and the nurse slipped the straw into my mouth. I exhaled deeply, then pulled strongly and steadily on the straw. The nurse's eyes widened as the level plummeted.

I worried momentarily about the quantity I had drunk, then thought, "What's a little sissy wine to a beer drinker with records to his name? Good old Harvey. Here's to him."

After half an hour my sensibilities slowly deserted me. Intellect first: I could no longer follow the professor's erudite discourse. "'Red nuclei,' did he say? I must be dreaming." Next, my hearing played tricks. Yes, Mozart had too many notes, no doubt about it.

I felt giddy and leaned against the operating table.

"Take a few deep breaths, Dick, you'll be O.K."

So I would have been but for my damn headlamp. My head felt odd. I stretched and my little light shone on the darkened ceiling where it wavered and danced like Tinkerbell. With an effort I pulled it down, whereupon it shone in the professor's eyes. When it finally returned to the operating field it flickered disconcertingly.

"Do you feel unwell?" the professor asked solicitously.

"I feel giddy, sir."

"He has postural hypotension," he declared, "due to pooling of blood in the lower extremities and a consequent fall in pressure. It is found in younger men"—smugly—"unaccustomed to prolonged standing. You may be excused," he said kindly, "we have only two more hours' work. I advise you do some brisk walking to restore normal circulation. Nurse, please assist him."

The assistance took the form of a violent prod as she ejected me from the room. I found sanctuary, collapsing in the doctors' changing room. We never had wine again and I never became a neurosurgeon.

Following a cerebral month of neurosurgery, Larry and I chose a manual task, a month of orthopedics. This enabled us to return to Central Middlesex, where a large number of trauma patients were admitted, mostly as a consequence of traffic accidents. They arrived at all hours so we decided to live in the hospital during the week. That enabled us to see and examine emergency cases as they were admitted, which is valuable.

Large hospitals make excellent hotels, for sustenance can be found at any hour either in the cafeteria or the ward kitchens. Sleeping is no problem as the residents' quarters house a shifting population and a bed is usually available. If not, one can be found on a ward, given an understanding nurse. Dress is simple. Scrub suits are adaptable for most tasks, a white coat can be added for formal occasions, and both items are cared for by the hospital laundry. Once you know the password you can make outgoing calls to your loved ones. All these amenities came at no charge, a major attraction.

Our new chief was an Australian who had been a brigadier during the war, serving in the Western Desert, Italy, and Germany. He was a tall, forbidding man, suited to be commandant of a detention barracks. At our first meeting he barked "Morton" and I responded instinctively by snapping to attention and producing a better salute than I had ever managed in the RAF. His specialty was, not unnaturally, trauma.

My spatial deficiency, which handicapped me in anatomy, also placed me at a disadvantage in orthopedics. I had one asset which he exploited—my strength. Orthopedics features a variety of devices—weights, pulleys, extenders—to position, stretch, turn, and immobilize the patient. These are heavy, tedious to assemble and adjust, particularly in the operating room. I proved to be a readily available alternative. While he and Larry operated, I elevated the leg, sometimes placing it on my shoulder or holding it in my cupped hands and moving on demand. I would pull steadily to hold a joint open or push to close it while they operated, sawing, nailing, and hammering away. When orthopedic topics staled, they reenacted the battle for Monte Cassino, interrupting only to direct me to pull harder, lift higher, or stand straighter. I needed no football training while on this rotation. When this strenuous and informative month came to an end, our teacher took us to a bibulous feast in a first-class restaurant, a welcome gesture which we much appreciated.

Larry suggested we attend a lecture on patient attitudes, which led to an unfortunate outcome. The major point was that patients are afraid of their doctors, and it was necessary for us to establish rapport with them, whereupon they would pour out their hearts' secrets. The method recommended for women was to enquire about their families; for men, about their work. These questions were not threatening, showed interest in them as individuals, and built rapport, which led to secrets revealed.

The suggestion appeared practical and I decided to follow it at the first opportunity, which arose the following morning when I was assigned a new patient. I had trouble locating him, for he was in a part of the hospital with which I was unfamiliar and so preoccupied was I with this new approach that I overlooked the first duty of the physician—observation. This would have told me that he was in the private wing, on the top floor, in the finest and most costly suite the hospital offered. On entering, I did not notice the sumptuous furniture nor did I study his chart. My patient was a man approaching seventy, white-haired, sitting erect in bed reading the *Times*, as dignified as one can be in a hospital gown. Fortunately, I omitted to introduce myself but opened the interview with my rehearsed question: "Hello, Pop, what did you do for a living?"

"I, Sir, am a High Court Judge." His expression implied that he regretted that he had not brought his "Black Cap" so that he could summarily sentence me to be dispatched at dawn. My patient was the only one in London not afraid of his doctor; on the contrary, the situation was reversed. Glancing at his chart I saw he was a Lord; worse, his doctor was also a Lord, past president of the Royal College of Surgeons. How should I address him? "My Lord?" "Your Lordship?" "Your Honor?" or just plain "Judge?" These were uncharted waters so I settled for the ubiquitous "Sir," and gathered a few facts about his illness. Any that proved to be missing I would improvise later. Signing my name illegibly, I scuttled out.

The surgical list revealed he was scheduled for a major procedure the next morning and I hoped he would have post-operative amnesia. I then persuaded Larry, who had got me into this predicament, to swap cases with me.

The last three of the six surgical months were spent in general surgery where I became dresser to Sir Robert, a pioneering surgeon who was developing a new, two-stage operation for cancer of the bowel, which combined abdominal incision with a pelvic approach. This was surgery on a grand scale and he was ideal for the task. Technically outstanding, he had an innovative mind together with perseverance, optimism, and confidence in his abilities. He was also inconsiderate, rude, and domineering. He was an icon and I was captivated, falling under his spell, a willing slave. This was all I imagined surgery would be; dramatic, tense, bloody, a battle of good against evil. The cancer could be seen and felt and Sir Robert schemed, maneuvered, and fought against it. It was eerie to look down from the abdominal wound and see his gloved hands appearing from below via the pelvic incision.

This was a juncture at which blood loss could be considerable and, in one instance, the anesthesiologist called suddenly for more blood. We had two lines open, one already with blood flowing, the pelvic one with fluid. The chief called, "Morton, break scrub, get some blood, put it in here quickly." At that time, blood was supplied in glass corked bottles. My gloves were greasy, and in my haste the open bottle slipped and fell into Sir Robert's surgical boot, filling it (glug, glug) to overflowing with 500 ccs of blood.

The operating room was Sir Robert's castle and he, in common with most surgeons, resented interruptions or, worse, intrusions. When closing incisions we sprayed a sulfonamide powder into them using bottles similar to ladies' cologne sprays. Once we were about to do this when both swing doors opened and the Brigadier, accompanied by a Bishop in full ecclesiastical regalia, including his hat, entered, unannounced and unwelcome. Before they could speak, our leader, holding his sprayer aloft, called: "Let us spray."

At the end of one long surgical day, a hemorrhoidectomy was added. This was a minor procedure. The chief told his assistant: "You go to the clinic. I'll do it." He should have left the minor to his junior and taken the clinic himself where more experience was needed, but it was not an appropriate moment to make this suggestion. The new patient, a large man, was wheeled in, drowsy from medication. The scrub nurse announced: "Anesthesia is all gone. It's late, sir, he wasn't listed. You'll have to wait for emergency anesthesia."

"'Wait'!" he expostulated. "Nothing but delay! I'll never get back to Harley Street this evening." (He did not really want to return to Harley Street or anywhere else—he wanted to stay, operating, in his beloved OR.)

"Anesthesia," he muttered scornfully, "man's as strong as a horse, why any fool—MORTON open the anesthesia pack, put a large line in, start some fluid. That's it—see the sodium pentothal, it's all made up, inject it in the side line, slowly now, that puts them to sleep. Clap the mask on his face, turn up the oxygen and nitrous oxide to the marks on the gauges. Good, let's get started. NURSE position him, that's right, now adjust the light."

Hemorrhoidectomy needs no assistant and only a few instruments. He dilated the anus, grasped the first hemorrhoid, pulling roughly. "AAGH!" cried the patient, jerking a leg and knocking over the instrument stand.

"MORTON give him some more pentothal, man, put him out! NURSE get up off the floor. Kick those instruments out of the way and fetch some clean ones. How can I work surrounded by incompetence?"

"How dare you move and ruin my best clerkship?" I addressed the patient silently. "Now he'll only remember me for this fiasco. I'll put you out so you won't wake up." I injected more pentothal. The patient became still. The operation was swiftly completed and the great man stalked out.

"He's left, thank God," said the nurse. "I'll clean up this mess if you'll put his legs down, they're heavy. We need a porter, but the porters have all gone. We'll never lift him—how will we get a porter?"

"Be quiet!" I shouted at her. "We don't need a porter, we need an anesthesiologist. This man is dead or close to it as far as I can tell. He can't breathe. Don't waste time, run to the anesthesia office and grab someone, anyone, or he's a goner and so am I."

She returned quickly with the chief of anesthesia. He promptly intubated the patient, better to ventilate him. "How much pentothal has he had?"

"Well, sir, I'm not quite—"

He broke in angrily. "What's happened here, who told you to give anesthesia?"

"This case was scheduled late, at 4:30 PM, sir. No anesthesia was available. The surgeon was told he must wait thirty minutes."

"You mean Sir Robert would have had to wait?" He reconsidered.

"So you were just following his orders? Luckily for all concerned and no thanks to you, this man will survive. Now follow my orders, which are that you will remain with him until he regains consciousness and can breathe on his own. Take his vital signs and record them every thirty minutes until they are stable, then do it hourly after that. One of us will visit through the night. I expect you will be there for twenty-four hours."

He was nearly correct, for it was eighteen hours before the patient finally woke up. His first words were: "Doc, that was wonderful, I never felt a thing."

In the summer of 1951 an opportunity presented for an obstetrics/gynecology rotation at a new location, a market town in Wales 215 miles west of London. I was the first incumbent and was housed in the hospital, which was small, but was the referral center, with consultants based there. The hospital was responsible for an area covering forty-five miles to the west, measuring thirty miles across and comprising two rural counties. The ocean formed the southern and western boundaries, girded by cliffs and headlands. In the interior were gently rolling wooded hills, with green pastures and meadows in the valleys. The fields were thick with waving yellow wheat, and cattle browsed on the hillsides. It was a welcome change from London.

Under the National Health Service, prenatal care was free of charge and available to all women. This excellent principle was cost-effective, insured good attendance, and provided screening early in pregnancy, which meant that women at high risk could be identified, treated, and delivered in special units. In this part of the U.K., the usual reasons for a woman to be considered at increased risk were previous obstetrical complications, a premature baby, or medical conditions that affect pregnancy. Factors such as drug use, excessive smoking and drinking, sexually transmitted diseases and, above all, poverty, were not as prevalent in these surroundings as they were in London.

— INDOCTRINATION —

The prenatal clinics were run by nurses, and midwives who were nurses with special training and certification delivered the babies. Doctors had only a consultant role and were called only in case of complications. Babies were born in bed, the patient lying on her side. Stirrups were used only in cases of difficult delivery, such as large babies, breech, or following prolonged labor. Forceps deliveries were uncommon, cesarean sections rare. Pain relief was given during labor, particularly for first babies, and the patients could use an inhaler that dispensed anesthetic and oxygen as they needed it. The atmosphere in the labor and delivery unit was friendly, relaxed, downright domestic. I spent a long time there at first, being taught by the midwives how to manage normal labor and delivery. My chief performed only the complicated deliveries—forceps, breech and a few cesarean sections.

In a prolonged labor, when it is vital to know the presentation of the head before applying forceps, the textbook method of feeling the bones of the fetal skull does not work, as they are soft and distorted by pressure. But the ear is a reliable marker, easily identified by feeling, and by wiggling it about you can tell which way the head is lying. My mentor showed me how to do this. He did not wear gloves, maintaining that they detracted from the sensitivity of the fingers.

Breech deliveries can be difficult and dangerous. The temptation is to pull on the protruding legs, which may severely damage the baby; hence, the maxim "hands off the breech." I was made to kneel on the floor when delivering a breech rather than standing or sitting. You look and feel stupid in that position but it lessens the desire to pull the legs, as the emerging baby is above you. When you have done this several times your experience teaches you that the mother will deliver the baby unaided if you merely guide it and refrain from pulling, which is awkward and unnatural when kneeling. In the few cases when spontaneous progress ceases, your instinct is not to pull but to investigate and remedy whatever is causing the delay.

In those days, patience in the delivery room was a virtue and was epitomized in the saying: "The stool is the most important instrument in the delivery room, for as long as you sit on it you won't do much damage." Today this type of management in a complicated delivery is an anachronism, but in 1951 it resulted in the best outcome for mother and baby.

— INDOCTRINATION —

The atmosphere in the operating room was relaxed, in contrast to London. Once surgery was under way, the anesthesiologist opened the *Times* newspaper and read aloud the Court Circular, which listed the engagements of the Queen and the Royal Family, in its entirety, followed by Church, Legal, and University appointments and promotions. The obituary page was scanned and my chief selected the entry to be read. I suspected he felt isolated in his rural setting and compensated by vicarious enjoyment of city life. Following the newspaper ritual, his secretary was summoned to the operating room, and the pair dealt efficiently with the mail. Two standards of notepaper were used, A and B. The former was for his superiors, peers and private patients, the latter for the remainder of his correspondents. His selection of A or B was decisive but occasionally he would dither; presumably, some subtle social factors were in fine balance.

Many of his letters were reports to doctors who had sent him complicated pregnancies and he used a stock phrase in concluding: "I know you will keep your eye on her." One replied: "I am returning her to you. I took my eye off her and she is pregnant again."

He first taught me D&Cs, known as dusting and cleaning, more formally as dilation and curettage of the uterus. Before starting I had to perform a pelvic examination under anesthesia and give him a verbal report. Then I had to record the size, shape, position, consistency and mobility of the uterus and ovaries, and any abnormal finding such as a tumor. This examination is the basic skill of a gynecologist, comparable to the auscultation of a cardiologist and special examination of a neurologist.

The pelvic architecture, seen from the abdominal approach (as contrasted with the vaginal), lends itself to teaching an assistant, for the structures are bilateral, identical on the right and left. I replaced the nurse and my teacher instructed me on my side of the table. The steps of any particular gynecological operation are simple to learn and perform. More important is to follow a routine in all cases. He taught me to feel all the accessible structures in the abdomen and pelvis and report on them when the operating field was first exposed. Once this has been done, one can focus on the pelvis. He operated in a deliberate, controlled manner, always in the same sequence, modified only by disease, be it tumor or infection. In a hysterectomy the blood vessels and ligaments of the uterus were each identified, dissected, and ligated in the same order. Such routine has much to commend it, which I did not appreciate until later when watching or assisting surgeons who lacked it. They would grab and claw at the uterus or ovary immediately the incision permitted it. They would do a little bit here, a little more there, fiddling about deep in the pelvis until the bleeding deterred them, avoiding the difficult dissection which should have been tackled first. By now it would be hazardous, the anatomy distorted and obscured by their haphazard efforts.

My chief was the first to introduce me to journals, as distinct from textbooks. He would select a disease such as diabetes, thyroid dysfunction, or multiple sclerosis and loan me a review article discussing the effects of the disease upon a pregnancy and vice versa. I was to read the textbook first, then the review and one or two articles cited in it. He encouraged me to use the journals in his library at home so that I could study one topic in depth, possible because, with no traveling or other distractions, I had more time here than in London. He operated five mornings a week, three in our hospital and two at smaller hospitals in other parts of his jurisdiction.

He and I inadvertently participated in a family drama. His wife was due to have their fourth child, delivery to be at home by the senior midwife. At 1:00 AM the telephone rang: "Morton, my wife is in labor. Inform Sister and accompany her to my house at once," he instructed me.

We left the hospital, hurried in the light of the moon past the pub, and crossed the road in the shadow of the War Memorial to reach his elegant home. He ushered us upstairs where his wife was lying in a large four-poster bed. The room was lit by one bedside light, which revealed that birth was clearly imminent. Sister clasped her patient's hand in greeting, then rapidly unpacked her bag.

"Is there anything you need?" asked the chief anxiously. More to occupy him than anything else, she replied, "More light would be welcome."

"Of course, I have the very thing, he replied. "Morton, come with me."

We hurried downstairs to his study in which he had recently installed a powerful standard light, better to illuminate his library shelves.

"Carry this please." We reappeared with our burden to find the midwife coaching the patient in breathing and relaxing as she approached the second stage of labor. I placed the lamp beside the bed and James bent down to plug it in. There followed a flash, an oath, and total blackness.

"James, dear, are you all right?"

"Dammit—oh, yes."

"I have a flashlight in my bag, sir, just a moment," interjected Sister. After some fumbling in the dark, a thin weak gleam appeared.

"Oh dear, I have only my penlight."

"James," came the authoritative voice of the patient between contractions, "go downstairs. On no account tamper with the fuses, I will summon the electrician in the morning. We need candles. They are in the kitchen, in the dry goods cupboard above the cereals but below the staples. That cupboard is between the broom closet and the tinned goods cupboard."

"The what," said my chief weakly.

"Baked beans, dear," she replied. "You will need matches. They are above the Aga on the left, beside the vent. Take care on the stairs, please. Oh!" A strong contraction supervened.

The house was old, with winding corridors and hidden steps. There were two staircases, the main flight and one in the back, which we took. The farmhouse kitchen was large, with obstacles scattered about—a big table, stools, and chairs. I struck my head on the ladles and saucepans that dangled from the ceiling. We located the Aga cooker by its warmth and I reached the precious matches.

"Quickly, open that cupboard, Morton."

I did so. It was full of bottles.

"Sir, we should follow directions. Let us locate the broom closet."

"Blast the brooms, open the next one."

It was clear that he was a stranger in his own kitchen. They had a cook and I doubted that he visited frequently. Matches flared and dazzled our eyes, then died and returned us to darkness.

"Sir, we should look for the baked beans."

"Bugger the beans, open that one." The cupboard contained packages, three of which fell out as I wrenched the door open. He snatched at one.

"Dammit, I've lost my glasses, what does this say?"

"Sago, sir."

"Sago? What the devil's that?"

"I'm not sure, sir, halfway between macaroni and spaghetti, I think." I reached down and picked up a large packet and shook it. It felt and sounded familiar. "Cornflakes here, sir."

"Stop talking and hurry!"

"Yes, sir, but more haste…"

"GET ON WITH IT!"

"Another match, please, sir. I have to reach above the cornflakes and shredded wheat—here are the candles."

He led the way upstairs, guided by the guttering candle. Upon re-entering the bedroom we knew at once all was well. No longer did his wife labor, her breathing was slow and regular and she lay back on the pillows with a serene expression, holding their baby. Her husband kissed her, murmuring endearments, still holding the candle. Sister relieved him of it and lit a second, placing both in holders.

I belatedly realized there was a large flashlight in his car, borrowed the penlight, and fetched it. Sister had cleared up and was saying goodbye. The mother said: "James, dear, you look exhausted. Please go to bed now in the spare room. Thank you all for your help. Baby and I will sleep until morning. Goodnight."

An itinerant Irish surgeon lived in the hospital. He wandered from one hospital to another, wherever he could find a job, always choosing rural sites. With the exception of some distant relatives in Eire, he had no family, home, or possessions, a dropout not willing to shoulder responsibilities or obligations either to people or institutions. He dealt with all emergencies, took all-night duty, ran a clinic, and spared the consultants many calls, and I suspected that they clubbed together to pay his salary. He would occasionally disappear, usually for a night, sometimes for a weekend. In these cases I deputized for him, for there was no one else to do so.

Faced with calls from patients he would suggest a variety of Gaelic remedies, recited in his Irish brogue, and at times I thought some called merely to sample his repertoire.

I assisted him at emergency surgery, usually in the small hours. This was enjoyable, but for one complication—he was having a torrid affair with the surgical night nurse. If she was scrubbed there were delays while they stared interminably into one another's eyes. If she was acting as circulating nurse the interruptions were longer. With the heat of the operating lights, compounded by the warmth of his passion, he sweated profusely and called frequently for a wipe, turning away from the table. She would then pull down his mask, tenderly wiping his sodden brow while they repeated the eye contact and heavy breathing routine. The anesthetist was almost as deeply asleep as the patient, but the second nurse and I were unwilling spectators to this lust, and I longed to suggest that we complete the operation as quickly as possible, following which they could enjoy consummation on the couch in the doctors' changing room.

Upon returning to London, I devoted a month to forensic medicine, which was lurid and intriguing. The textbook featured a picture of a headless corpse captioned, "Foul play suspected," together with the comment, "Police are anxious to interview the husband of the deceased, hoping he will be able to assist them in their inquiries."

Graduation was due in May and I procrastinated until April before making any plans to emigrate to the U.S. Belatedly, I visited their embassy, requesting an interview with the chief medical officer.

The embassy staff had cross-cultural confusion. The clerical employees, whom I first encountered, pretended to be Americans, adopting what they imagined were U.S. accents, idioms, mannerisms, and dress. I knew they were, like me, Londoners by origin. They knew I knew but persisted, for practice I presume. My request was unusual so eventually I was interviewed by two members of the consular staff, who were Americans. They, in turn, masqueraded as English aristocrats and I, pretending to be convinced by their performance, responded in kind so we chaps had a jolly chat.

Finally, the interview was granted. The doctor behaved normally, secure in his identity with no role reversal, and so, with relief, did I. I modestly asked which was the finest hospital in America. He replied that the honors were evenly divided between Massachusetts General Hospital (MGH: Man's Greatest Hospital) in Boston, and Johns Hopkins Hospital in Baltimore. Asked to select one, he replied that it depended on the specialty in which I was seeking training. Informed that it was ob/gyn he said Hopkins was the choice, for Dr. Eastman, author of the standard textbook, was chief of obstetrics and Dr. TeLinde, author of another standard work, was chief of gynecology. He then consulted a directory, which revealed that only six places were offered every year by each chief. For these vacancies over one hundred well-qualified Americans would apply and a foreign medical graduate (FMG)—the first time I heard this unpleasant term—stood no chance of acceptance. He recommended that I read the advertisements in the Journal of the American Medical Association, where a section was reserved for FMGs. He explained that the vacancies were all for rotating internships in small hospitals, most of them in rural states, and recommended that I apply to all as the best chance to secure one. This kind and practical advice came from a graduate of the Harvard University School of Medicine and of their medical residency program at MGH, as evidenced by the certificates in his office.

He concluded our meeting by giving me the current issue of JAMA and his best wishes, adding that I was the first English doctor to have consulted him on emigration. I felt sobered, crestfallen and uncertain, and that my ambition was impractical and foolish. Surely it would be wiser to apply for an internship at Middlesex, where the training would surpass that of a small, non-teaching hospital in the U.S.? Internships were difficult to get at Middlesex, being reserved for honor students, whereas I was mediocre. But the chief of radiotherapy had played rugby as a forward for Australia, knew me, and was known to employ large rugby players. Unfortunately, I wanted to go into ob/gyn, not radiotherapy.

A major problem was that we planned to marry immediately upon my graduation and if I went to a small hospital in rural America, would Kate ever join me there? It would not have been fair to ask her, for she was an honor student and would be offered a medical internship at the Middlesex. A compromise would be to train in England and then go to America together four years later, but I feared postponement would be fatal. Disconsolately, I meandered my way from the splendid embassy in Mayfair to seedy Soho, where I settled in the hospital library intending to read the JAMA. As I passed the list of medical lectures to be delivered in London, a name caught my eye. Dr. Eastman, obstetrician of Johns Hopkins, would talk at Guy's Hospital the following day.

At the lecture, which attracted a number of prominent obstetricians, it became evident that Dr. Eastman was an anglophile. He was called "Nick" by his hosts and friends, and it was clear that he felt at home in England.

He had chosen for his topic "the management of premature rupture of the membranes." When this common complication occurs, the fetus is immediately in jeopardy both from infection and from preterm labor. The outcome for the baby depends primarily on the length of the pregnancy; the shorter it is, the worse the result. Treatment varied from watchful waiting to immediate cesarean section. No consensus prevailed—each case was handled individually according to the judgment and experience of the doctor in charge. Some hospitals published small series of cases purporting to justify the conservative or the radical approach.

Dr. Eastman's discussion differed fundamentally from any I had previously read or heard, for it was entirely numerate. The obstetrical records at Hopkins were standardized, detailed, and complete. When they were subsequently analyzed, the results, in terms of fetal survival, could be tabulated, cross-classified, examined, and displayed in a variety of ways. His survey included a large number of cases dating back many years. Shown in colored slides, a novelty at that time, they demonstrated that the length of gestation (i.e., the maturity of the pregnancy) was the dominant factor governing outcome, regardless of the method of treatment. But, broken down into periods of gestation—early, intermediate and mature—the differing effects of treatment could be discerned in each group. The influence of infection could be singled out by comparing those so threatened with those that were not, indicating that infection worsened the outcome in every case. This method enabled like to be compared with like, with confounding factors controlled.

It was clear that the majority of the audience found this numerical approach uncongenial, compared with the clinical discussions to which they were accustomed. Too polite to criticize an overseas visitor harshly, they cited single cases from their experience that contradicted a conclusion reached from the group data, not realizing that this was inevitable given the nature of probability. Although it is correct to base management on the findings demonstrated from the majority of cases rather than the exceptions, this was alien to the clinicians, who naturally rely on their individual experience.

I decided to write to Dr. Eastman, on the principle of "nothing ventured, nothing gained." Managing to be brief, I related how I had enjoyed his lecture, particularly the detailed analysis of a large series of cases. I confessed to experiencing a revelation; namely, that obstetrics lends itself to enumeration, as the same sequence of events is repeated innumerable times. I then explained that following graduation in May I hoped to work for him as an intern. I steeled myself for the probability of no reply or, at best, a routine rejection letter, as I had delayed too long (a Freudian slip, perhaps, signifying that I really did not wish to leave England). I tried to forget about the letter, which was made easier by the need to concentrate on the exams that were soon approaching. Should I fail any of these, my problems would be over. Then, two weeks later, in the middle of breakfast, Mother brought in the mail and announced, "A letter from Baltimore for you, dear." As she handed me a small envelope with the Hopkins Dome insignia embossed on heavy white bond paper, eggs and bacon turned to ashes in my mouth, and I could not bring myself to open it at the table before my parents. Since the envelope was small, no application form could be enclosed, just a rejection. I excused myself, went up to my room, and slit open the envelope: "Dear Mr. Morton. Thank you for your letter. I have long wished to employ an Englishman but hitherto none has applied. Please arrange an interview with Dr. _____ (naming the chief of ob/gyn at Guy's, his recent host) and then report to my office on June 30, 1953, prepared to serve as an intern for six months in obstetrics followed by six in gynecology. Yours sincerely, Nicholson J. Eastman. P.S. You may encounter some initial minor statutory problems."

I had done it but felt overwhelmed and weak. Returning to the kitchen, I passed the letter to Father. Glancing at it, he said, "Good, a job," and resumed reading the newspaper, while Mother, sad as she was, embraced me. My brother had left for the U.S. two years previously. Mother would be left with no children to spoil.

The interview at Guy's was fraught with unexpressed thoughts and prejudices on both sides. The purpose was to confirm that I was what I purported to be. This my interlocutor could ascertain by a telephone call, which I believed he had already made. He posed some desultory questions about my training but competence was not in question, it would be measured by the forthcoming examinations. From his attitude I realized that he found emigration distasteful, that leaving for America and capitalizing on the education vouchsafed me by England was defection, a venal act, mercenary in character, unworthy of a gentleman, and that he despised me for it. He tried valiantly but failed to mitigate his evident dislike of me. Being English, we did not mention our differences but masked them and

I had no fear that he would prejudice me in a report, for his sobriquet was "Honest John."

The final examinations were, like medical practice, an endurance test. Each subject, of which there were six, contained a written, clinical, and oral component. The written occupied the first week, the remainder a second week. The University of London took the wise precaution of ensuring that the students of one hospital should be examined in the wards of another. The logistics of this, in pre-computer days, posed a challenge for the examiners, patients, and seven hundred students, all of whom had to meet at prearranged times and locations. We were the mobile element so we dashed about London from one hospital to another. Forty-five minutes were allotted for a long case and fifteen for a short, during which a history and physical examination had to be performed and the results discussed with the examiner.

An identification parade of patients with conditions that could be diagnosed by one salient feature was a renowned hazard. Examiners prowled about a large hall and pounced upon a student barking, "Examine this man's left eye. What is this skin condition? Identify this patient's gait. What is the cause of this withered arm?" Two examiners questioned us for fifteen minutes in each of the six oral exams; it seemed forever to us and probably to them.

I had no special dread such as that which had threatened me in anatomy three years previously. I wanted only to pass and was not seeking distinction, for which I was not fitted, and due to good fortune I had already secured the internship I sought. I concentrated on my weak areas, neglecting the few strong ones.

On one occasion, I was fortunate when wandering around St. Bartholomew's, one of the oldest hospitals in England. Searching for the right ward, I came to a back staircase at the foot of which stood an elderly lady with a suitcase. "Let me carry that for you," I volunteered, "I'm looking for the cardiology ward."

"Thank you," she replied, "I'll show you the way, I know it only too well." We climbed several flights slowly, in companionable silence. On arrival, I had to wait, then was summoned to the long medical case, which was my new friend. Showing no sign of recognition, she whispered her diagnosis and sundry valuable information to me.

Events now moved swiftly. On May 13, 1953, Kate's twenty-second birthday, the exam results were posted. We decided to marry at once and made an appointment at the Marylebone Registry Office, four blocks north of the hospital, for May 15. Our news was received coolly by our families. Fortunately, little time was left for preparation and we had no money, which simplified matters.

I forked out seven shillings and sixpence for a license ($1.50), the best investment I ever made. One of Kate's many friends was the photographer employed by pathology, based in the morgue, who volunteered to take the pictures provided we remained "very, very still."

A posy of lilies of the valley which I bought for her were the only flowers and doubled as a wedding gift. Eight guests attended, all family, the oldest of whom was Kate's grandfather, "Pop." He used to rise at 5:00 AM daily and greet each sunrise with a bottle of beer. On this day, Kate was up early and, once he grasped that it was her wedding day, he continued greeting the sun, with the result that he was drunk, though not disorderly, at the brief ceremony.

Once we were married and stood (very still) on the steps of the Town Hall, Kate holding my arm, I felt twice the man. Terence, my father-in-law, had a gift, lunch in the Grill Room of the Savoy Hotel, a spontaneous gesture that was typical of him and which afforded us our first, and only, visit there.

Our wedding was modest by any standard, our reception was not since it was piggy-backed on to the Hospital Ball. This annual event was organized by a student committee of which Kate was chair, having been the first woman elected to that office. Driving home across Waterloo Bridge earlier in the year we had been discussing the Ball and where it should be held.

"People are bored with hotels," Kate had said, "why don't we hold it there?" as she waved at Festival Hall, a new building that had just opened. It enjoyed an attractive site at the south end of Waterloo Bridge, providing a fine view of the London skyline and river Thames.

"Don't be silly," I responded, "it's for symphonies and concerts, not dances."

"I'm going to ask anyway. They may consider a charity ball attractive."

— INDOCTRINATION —

Her committee members, all male, concurred with my negative reaction but feminine intuition proved correct. The Festival Hall had never considered hosting a Ball but as the proceeds were to benefit a charity and 500 luminaries of the medical establishment would attend, it became available. Society press coverage was assured, mutually advantageous to the Hospital and Festival Hall, so it proved to be a marriage made in heaven.

Thus, our marriage, made in Marylebone, was celebrated that evening at the Hospital Ball. Kate changed from her blue wedding suit to a long gown, I from my only suit to a tuxedo, and we drove to the Hall, top down and spirits up. All agreed it was a festive occasion and Kate was feted for her initiative in securing the venue and also for her marriage to a Middlesex man (any of whom would have done).

The Hall rose to the occasion. A chamber music ensemble that had just concluded performing was ousted in favor of a dance orchestra. The concertgoers, conservatively clad and sober, left, to be replaced by the medical elite, who were dressed to the nines and full of bonhomie. The consultants had organized private dinner parties and they were ready to mingle and dance. The premises were gaily decorated, with extra bars added at strategic spots. We students, who had just passed our finals, were in high spirits, and our juniors were encouraged by our success, correctly believing that if we could pass so could they. I said goodbye to my teachers, team and classmates. We walked on the terrace by moonlight, watching the silhouette of London across the river, and "Oh, how we danced on the night we were wed." Time passed on gilded wings and, as the sparrows awoke, we drove home.

We left London the same day, driving to Wales, where we would spend our honeymoon. Kate had arranged a medical rotation at the hospital and I resumed the training that I had enjoyed the previous summer. We rented a room in a cottage beside the hospital but no telephone was available so, in order that I could be reached at night, I wore a cord with a weight attached around my wrist which led out of the window down to the ground. In response to a persistent tugging on the cord, I would raise the window and, looking down, see a student nurse in a uniform with leg-of-mutton sleeves peering up. "Hurry, Doctor, you're needed." Disentangling myself from my communications equipment and donning a scrub suit, I would reach the delivery rooms quickly. The night staff managed the majority of births and were sparing in calling me. That we were newlyweds was hardly a secret. We had chosen Wales, their town and hospital for our honeymoon, so that almost excused us for being English and Londoners.

Women behaved differently in Soho compared with women in rural Wales. In Soho they were generally treated as social equals to men—and this was certainly true in pubs—but in Wales their status was lower. Women rarely entered pubs and then only in a special bar, never the saloon. The pub was conveniently situated opposite the hospital and I was known from my previous visit. Despite this, when Kate and I first entered the saloon bar together the reaction was inhospitable and we felt that we had committed some infraction.

Kate was young, tall, blonde, dressed in black trousers. Her voice was clear and very English. She was confident and when a man glared at her she responded with, "Hello, how are you tonight?" In a word not then used, she was assertive. Two brothers ran the pub but it was owned by their aunt, to whom I introduced Kate. Auntie gave her ready acceptance and moral support, making it clear she was welcome in the saloon. It was my first experience of the sisterhood in action and very effective it was.

My mentor had arranged a meeting for me with a retired chief of obstetrics who lived at Laugharne, a village notorious because the poet Dylan Thomas lived there. My host was in his nineties—spry, alert, all faculties sound. He demonstrated some old obstetrical instruments in his library and asked: "Have you done any symphysiotomies?" to which I replied, "No, sir." This operation, a forerunner of cesarean section, entailed splitting the front joint between the two halves of the pelvis, left and right, which permitted vaginal delivery, otherwise impossible, and prevented certain fetal death with serious maternal complications. The price paid was that the joint would not heal, resulting in a permanent scissors gait. He commented, "An unsatisfactory operation but you can always recognize your patients."

Laugharne is situated on an estuary and at ebb tide a wide stretch of beach is uncovered. In the afternoon sun, we walked on the ribbed sand.

"Hear you're going to Hopkins?"

"Yes, sir."

"Osler's there, isn't he?"

"He was, sir," I replied. Dr. Osler, the first and foremost of the four physicians who founded the John Hopkins University School of Medicine, later became Professor of Medicine at Oxford University. He had died in 1927.

The doctor continued, "I called him in twice, the first time to see a patient with childbed fever. He examined her, made some suggestions, but she died. The second case was a laborer who developed heart failure, she also died. Didn't ask him again." Looking out over the ocean he exclaimed, "Medicine is a race. I am flagging and hand the baton to you."

The coronation of Queen Elizabeth was celebrated. Bonfires were built on the hills and processions held. My parents visited, staying at a nearby ocean resort, where we joined them for a weekend. Pendine Sands, a long, lonely beach, provided a site for sunbathing and walks, and these numbered days, bittersweet, quickly passed. Separation hung over us, for after six weeks of marriage, sixteen months lay between my departure and Kate's graduation.

Kate chose to move into my house, for only my parents were living there. The four of us were a melancholy party as we drove to Southampton and, from the deck of the *Île de France,* my heart was in turmoil as I waved goodbye to Kate, my parents and England.

Chapter 4

Under the Dome

I was leaning on the starboard bow rail of the ship at dawn when the shore came into view, the New York City skyline sparkling in the sun. New York flaunts herself, standing boldly at the water's edge, not concealed for miles up an estuary like Washington and London. A colorful moving stream puzzled me—yellow, red, blue, green, white, flashing along—what could that be? As we neared the shore I discerned that they were automobiles speeding along the Shore Road. Cars in England were dull and dirty, usually black, with some blue or green permitted. They were small, for the roads are narrow and winding, and people drove slowly for the same reasons. Here the scale was larger, the pace quicker. That was clear even to an offshore observer.

As an alien traveling third class, I waited in line. The immigration officer bellowed, "Name?" The man in front of me replied, "Swiderski." The official wrote this down unerringly. To my response, "Morton," he demanded, "Spell it." Upon landing on U.S. soil I was encumbered by two heavy suitcases but little cash. To conserve the latter I walked to the bus terminal, having been advised that Greyhound offered the cheapest means of reaching Baltimore.

The contrast between Manhattan and London was striking. The colors here were bright and garish, not gray and staid. The inhabitants were dressed for the summer weather, whereas Londoners would have remained in suits and ties, carrying raincoats. The variety and abundance in the stores were amazing to me after the restricted offerings in London, and the rewards of success were visible, tangible and enticing. The bus, whose size and speed impressed me, roared through the tunnel toward the delights of New Jersey. The oil refineries were my first intimation of the industrial strength of the U.S., calling to mind a Yorkshire saying, "Where there's muck there's money."

We traveled the New Jersey Turnpike, unlike any road I had ever experienced, and when we made a stop at a Howard Johnson's the menu overwhelmed me—twenty-nine varieties of ice cream! At home, vanilla was the staple; occasionally, chocolate, and rarely, strawberry, were available. My fellow travelers ordered quickly and precisely. "Pistachio, hold the nuts." "Vanilla, heavy on the fudge!" "Coffee, plenty of sprinkles." I pored over the menu, and the waitress called, "Hurry up, Mac, choose or quit." "Chocolate, please," I replied, and barely made it back to the bus.

As the journey resumed, I became despondent, fearing that Hopkins would be all theory, biochemistry, laboratory tests and lectures. My ignorance would subject me to ridicule and disgrace. I tried, and failed, to recall what little I knew of obstetrics as a science, as opposed to an art.

We crossed the Susquehanna River as it terminated in Chesapeake Bay and then, as the song goes, "We were in Baltimore." It was afternoon on June 30. The city was hot and humid and my thick English woolen clothes unsuitable. Carrying the suitcases, I walked through the city and up the long hill to the hospital, arriving soaked in sweat.

The Johns Hopkins Hospital stands on a fifty-five-acre island site east of and above the city, looking downtown to the west and over the harbor to the south. On entering the building from Broadway you are confronted by a heroic twelve-foot marble statue of Christ dominating a small rotunda of six stories, above which stands the Dome, reached by a broad staircase. The hospital has been compared to a temple—a good analogy, as it is a large building on a hill, capped by a dome, containing a chapel and a statue of a god. All the elements found in temples are present. Priests in white robes are served in turn by acolytes and handmaidens. The premises, decorated with flowers, are crowded with supplicants seeking deliverance. The Hindu and Buddhist pagodas I had visited in India, Ceylon and Burma were similar: people and animals lived in them, and food and drink could be found in addition to spiritual guidance. These Asian buildings were surrounded by stalls selling gifts for pilgrims to leave in the temple as tributes. Similar shops nestled beside the hospital.

My room, shared with two other interns, was at the top immediately under the Dome. No elevators sullied this, the oldest part of the hospital. Walking further revealed a courtyard similar to the one in the Middlesex

Hospital. Turning left brought me to a dining room marked "Doctors," of which I made a special note.

Beyond this lay the main artery of the hospital, a wide corridor that stretched the length of the building. It was heavily trafficked with nurses and young doctors walking swiftly along the sides, their seniors in white coats pursuing a leisurely course in the center, all interspersed with patients and hospital employees. The specialties were clearly indicated along this corridor: medicine, surgery, pediatrics, urology, radiology, pathology. There was no evidence of obstetrics or gynecology and I emerged through the back door, reaching the street at the rear of the hospital opposite the School of Public Health. The only other missing discipline was psychiatry. Perhaps both were exiled to some hidden corner between the furnace, garbage and laundry.

Too weak to carry my suitcases any further, I was retreating back through the dingy exit I had just left when I noticed a small sign stating, "Women's Clinic." That no money had been spent on advertising, decoration, or vainglory was obvious and it later became plain that no money was spent, period—particularly on interns.

I was directed to a room where about twenty people were assembled. I sat at the back while my new chief, Dr. Eastman, presided. A resident was describing a pregnancy, labor and delivery of a dead baby. When the session was over he greeted me, inquiring if I had enjoyed the discussion. I confessed that it was my first experience of a fetal mortality conference, as in England only a maternal death merited such inquiry. Dr. Eastman, who commanded a vivid phraseology replied, "Maternal mortality can be prevented. Today the spotlight is on the fetus. The obstetrician shall become pediatrician to the fetus." In this, as in many obstetric topics, he was accurate and twenty years ahead of his time.

The tools necessary to reduce maternal mortality, such as advances in anesthesiology, blood and fluid replacement, treatment of infection, and rapid transport of the seriously ill to regional centers, had all been developed during the war. Now, eight years later, these improvements had resulted in a swift fall in deaths from pregnancy and childbirth. This decrease had not been uniform across states and within cities. True, all women had participated in the benefit, but the dispossessed and disadvantaged still, as always, had higher rates than their more fortunate sisters. To correct this iniquity, political action was, and still is, required.

I started to carry my suitcases up the six long flights to the Dome when a stranger volunteered to help me, who proved to be a gyn resident in his first year. Dwain had just returned from two years as a medical officer in the Korean War, and had driven from his home in Minnesota. I offered to assist him with his baggage, which comprised a carful of clothes, books, and sports equipment. We reached his old but well-preserved Chevrolet, which was parked on the street fronting the psychiatry building, only to find it empty. Everything had been stolen during the few minutes when he had been helping me. I attempted to console him, explaining that food and uniforms were provided and that these were all he would need.

Later, the six obstetric interns met; three Americans and three foreigners, reflecting Dr. Eastman's global view of medicine. Citing name, hometown, and undergraduate and medical schools our lineup read: Mark, Atlanta, Princeton, Emory; Maurice, Cleveland, Harvard, Harvard; Steve, Memphis, University of Virginia, Duke; José, Guadalajara, Columbia, New York, Mexico City; Dey, The Hague, Cambridge University, Leiden, and myself. We were all males. I never saw any female house staff but there were a few women consultants, the same low proportion as in London. The two southerners were married and I, at twenty-nine, was the oldest.

We had just introduced ourselves when a resident, a year senior to us, arrived to brief us. He explained the schedule, which was simple. We were on duty for twenty-four hours every Monday, Wednesday, Saturday, Sunday, Tuesday, Thursday, and Friday in each two-week period. On the days we were "off" we only worked from 7:00 AM to 8:00 PM except on Saturday, when we concluded at 1:00 PM Alternate Sundays were free. As he described it I figured we worked 230 hours every fourteen days, or sixty-eight percent on duty.

The three duty locations were the labor and delivery floor, the clinics, and the emergency room. We would spend a month in each site, then repeat the process. Coincident with this, we were to staff the in-patient beds, which were divided into pre- and post-delivery wards. There followed a long list of laboratory duties, including typing and cross-match-ing blood, the latter alarming me since all I knew was that there are four blood types and, that as with wine, one should not mix them. During the introduction our three natives all produced notebooks and pencils and efficiently inscribed the instructions that were flowing over us. We three aliens looked bewildered until our senior took pity and assured us that "it would all become clear as we went along." The session concluded with a few housekeeping matters. We were to be issued clothing, white coats and pants for dress uniform and scrub suits for battle fatigues, and the hospital would launder them at no charge. All meals were to be taken in the doctors' dining room at no charge, and supper, at 7:00 PM, was about to be served. He left after giving us our first assignments, whereupon Steve from Memphis remarked, in his southern drawl, "Ah hope that's all clear to you boys."

What was clear was that in order to last we all had to help one another, which we did, unstintingly, throughout the year. I attribute our survival to this cooperation. We obstetric interns finished the course with no illness or absence, whereas one intern withdrew from gynecology after six months and had to be replaced.

No mention had been made of vacation or pay, for there was none of either. No pay was the first of the "minor statutory problems" described by Dr. Eastman in his letter. I put it out of my mind and it proved of scant consequence as I had neither time nor energy for any diversion that required money.

My first assignment was the emergency room, where I noticed several black women lying on stretchers in the corridor. I had never cared for a black patient before, I could not read the scribbled notes of my predecessor who had disappeared, and I felt at a loss.

As I wondered where to start and what to do, I noticed one patient lying with her knees drawn up, occasionally turning them from side to side. This posture is adopted by patients with pelvic pain, frequently due to peritonitis and/or intra-pelvic bleeding. Reaching her side I heard her moaning quietly. I pulled over a blood pressure machine and while fitting the cuff inquired when her last menstrual period had been. She replied softly that she didn't rightly know as it was late, had started, stopped, started again but didn't seem regular. Then the pains had begun low down and had suddenly gotten worse.

She was thin and I put my hand gently on her lower belly. She guarded, tensing her muscles and trying to push my big hand away with her small one. Her pelvis was tender and I felt there was distension. I tried to take her blood pressure, but not hearing anything thought the machine was broken or that my stethoscope had not survived the journey. After exhorting myself to calm down and pull myself together I heard a soft systolic, low, about sixty. Her eye mucosa was pale, her pulse rapid and weak.

I said to the nurse, "This patient has a ruptured ectopic and is in shock. Get some saline and an eighteen needle, what's the number of labor and delivery, thanks." Despite not recognizing my name the resident responded quickly and the patient was taken to the operating room.

Later, Dr. Eastman complimented me. This was the only time I distinguished myself during my time at Hopkins and I had to waste it on the first day.

The month in the ER provided a cultural introduction to the patients for me, as listening to them compelled me to understand their idiom. In describing their reproductive histories they resembled their London counterparts but differences appeared in descriptions of their symptoms. My questions were couched in unfamiliar terms so I learned to ask fewer and listen more, a needed improvement. With menstrual data, misunderstandings occurred at first. Questioning a large lady who complained of excessive bleeding I asked, "Have you had a heavy loss before?" She considered carefully then responded proudly, "I once lost ten pounds."

The only place we worked that was air-conditioned was the ER, so when on night duty I slept there between calls, lying on a stretcher in the cool hall. The alternative was to climb six flights to my bed in a stifling room, lie down and expect to be recalled to work shortly. The ER was busier in the summer than in the winter, attracting a wide range of pathology, trauma, and homicide. We had to write complete histories in a specific order, an excellent practice but time-consuming, and sometimes I fell asleep at the desk, pen in hand. I recall one kind patient gently squeezing my hand to wake me, so when I opened my bleary eyes they were staring into her brown ones. She said, "Doc, you're exhausted, you need your rest. I've been resting too on that table, watching you sleep. I feel better now so I'll go on home, you go back to sleep."

One night during my first week I saw a patient with unusual menstrual problems whom I thought should be admitted for study. I consulted the roster to find that Al, a Canadian, the chief gyn resident, was on call. To marshall my facts I had all the dates and symptoms written down and at 2:30 AM I called. He answered at the first ring. "Al, Dick calling from the ER. This patient has an interesting history. Now she's... " I reeled out dates and symptoms but Al made no response and listening carefully I could hear his regular breathing—he was asleep.

I hung up, dialed again—busy. I found his address and asked the nurse for directions and was told: 1) I was forbidden to go out, 2) it was dangerous to go there at this hour. I rushed out anyway and located the small row house but before I had rung the bell the door shook and thunderous barks sounded. I, in common with most Englishmen, like dogs and am a large dog specialist. This was fortunate. As the door opened, I said softly, "Good boy, love you," whereupon Brutus, a five-year-old, 180-pound Great Dane, put his paws on my shoulders and began to lick my face fervently. Al's wife at first tried to dislodge him but while he was washing me he wasn't barking, so we conducted our interview in this stance. "Al was asleep," she said, apologizing, "did the patient have an immediate surgical indication?"

"No."

"Or a critical medical condition? No? Then give her an early clinic appointment," this diplomatic woman advised me. Brutus and I parted reluctantly and I promised him I would take him for a walk. When I asked permission from Al he was surprised that I knew he had a Dane. Thereafter, when I could get away from the hospital for a brief time I walked with Brutus, unmolested, through Patterson Park or down to the harbor. This rent-a-dog arrangement worked well for all parties.

When first living among Americans during the war I had found them friendly and hospitable, and this remained true. On my first free Saturday afternoon a gyn resident said, "I was born here, let me show you the town." We visited landmarks while he told me of the history of Baltimore, and then stopped downtown at Cushner's Men's Store, which he strode into as if he owned it. "You need some summer clothes now and something for later," he commanded. I was fitted with a tropical suit, shirts, and accessories, including a Panama. A darker, heavier weave for the lovely fall and spring seasons Baltimore offers was added, with shirts and ties to match. He found a pair of size thirteen white shoes, saying, "You can't wear those old sneakers to rounds any more. You're letting the side down, old boy."

He then introduced me to his father, who did own the store, and who said, "Irv has chosen some fancy clothes but I'm going to give you something that will last." To my surprise he fetched a felt hat in a smart hue with a colorful feather. I had not worn a hat since leaving the RAF. "As you grow older," he explained, "you'll need a hat in the cold weather." He showed me how to brush it, care for it and store it. I wore his hat for thirty-seven years, more frequently as time passed, as he predicted.

Leaving the store, carrying parcels of merchandise, I protested, "Irv—Irv, I can't pay you for this," to which he replied, "No, you certainly can't," and would hear nothing further on the subject.

Thirty-three years later, when I was visiting Los Angeles from New York, he invited me to the large city hospital where he was chief of obstetrics. I enjoyed making ward rounds and meeting the residents, the majority of whom were women.

We did not discuss medicine at dinner. Seated at a window table, high up, looking over the carpet of twinkling lights that is Los Angeles at night, we talked of old friends and old times. Irv was tired, still in the front line from which I had retreated, ostensibly to study the larger picture. We said goodbye in the warm fragrant Californian night. I never saw him again. He died the following week.

The dining room at Hopkins served as a social center, because we had no common room or lounge. The tables, seating ten, were all circular as at King Arthur's court, so we knights were all equal. The specialties sat together as it was necessary to conduct business as well as conversation, but several of the faculty joined us at meals, which leavened the mix.

Johns Hopkins harbored some peculiar characters—idiosyncratic, maverick, talented, but odd. They were not numbered among the great, never chairmen of a department, division or even a committee. They were secreted in closets, labs, corners, basements, and attics, and only two or three others in the hospital, indeed the university, knew, let alone understood, what they were doing. But they were prized, and their chairmen would fight to retain them. Since this was before the era of federal subsidies for research, they labored for love.

I recall visiting the worksites of three such unheralded scientists. One grew and sustained the line of cervical cancer cells named Hela, all harvested originally from one patient. The second worked in cytology and developed the techniques that enabled cervical (Pap) smears to be interpreted and graded into degrees of pathological significance.

The third, Charles, who became my friend, worked in obstetrics as a fetal and placental pathologist, the first of his kind. Dr. Eastman recognized that in order for the obstetrician to become pediatrician to the fetus, the interface between it and the mother, namely the placenta, must be studied and fetal pathology clarified. Charles was his nominee for this task.

I learned that Charles was an erudite man, an authority on the Revolutionary and Civil Wars, about which I knew little. Like other Americans of his class he had an ambivalent view of the British, outwardly derisive, almost hostile, yet with hidden admiration bordering on envy of some elements of British heritage. Hearing my voice at mealtimes he must have thought Fate had delivered to him a hostage, a renegade Englishman who had renounced Queen, country, birthright and bride to sup at the bountiful table of one of the erstwhile colonies.

He opened his campaign by asking if Cornwallis was a typical English commander. Military history happened to be the only branch of the discipline in which I was interested, and my scant knowledge was limited to World Wars I and II. I sparred with him and we had enjoyable exchanges, which he usually won. Extending the discussion to current American politics he would observe sardonically, "They order these matters better in the Mother of Parliaments, I presume?"

"Indubitably, they do, with debate that transcends any to be heard in Congress," I would reply. These wordy debates were becoming tedious to others at table, and sensing this he invited me to accompany him on some of his trips to nearby historic battlefields. Through the year on a few of my free weekends, we journeyed pleasurably together in his old jalopy.

As our intimacy grew he lifted a corner of the curtain behind which he sheltered. He lived alone in a room opposite the hospital, but he took most of his meals with us. Work was his passion, history his hobby and the bottle his weakness. It would tempt him rarely but when it did it brought complete surrender. In a section of downtown Baltimore called the Block were a cluster of tawdry bars and strip tease joints. Occasionally, we received a call from friends or acquaintances who knew he was connected to obstetrics that Charles was on the Block. We then assembled a posse of two or three, located him and, with a mixture of inveiglement and coercion, brought him home. He was literally taken away by men in white coats for his own good.

Our parting in June was fraught with unspoken concerns on both sides. He knew what awaited me in New York but spared telling me. I was worried that when the reign of Dr. Eastman terminated his successor might not appreciate Charles's contributions as much as Dr. Eastman had and he would have to move. Events proved me correct but I was pleased to hear that Charles had found a congenial home in a large obstetric hospital in New England.

The Middlesex was managed by our teachers, the consultants. They determined the diagnosis and treatment of all the patients, performed the major surgery and directed the clinics. Hopkins was different. The residents ran the hospital. They controlled admissions, made the diagnoses and prescribed treatment, and performed all the surgery—assisted, in major cases, by their chiefs. Patients admitted to obstetrics frequently had medical problems; heart disease, hypertension, diabetes, pulmonary disease, anemia, alcoholism, and a variety of other, less common, conditions. As interns, we cared for the whole patient and her disease in addition to rendering prenatal care or pre- and post-operative treatment. We asked our senior residents for guidance when needed and they decided if consultation from medicine or another service was indicated, which rarely proved to be the case. Our program was a "straight internship" in contrast to the majority in other hospitals where the intern rotates through the year in four or more different departments. Though our concentration was on ob/gyn we did not lack for training and experience in medicine.

The senior resident in every department at Hopkins was omnipotent and a clash between him and the chairman would have provoked a constitutional crisis. However, this was unlikely for the senior was the survivor of extensive culling of his peers by the chairman; he was thus honed to the latter's specifications. The senior residents had all worked five years at Hopkins and many in the subspecialties for seven or eight. The residency system was superior to the English model, for it provided graduated responsibility as one advanced, together with excellent teaching from peers. It also raised morale and fostered pride and comradeship among the group, as in the Marines (once a Marine, always a Marine) or the old regiments in the British Army (You're not in the Army, you're in the Guards).

Fortunately, many worries are unfounded and so it proved with my concern over my lack of science. Science I am sure there was, but it never percolated down to my level. I was taught clinically, in coinage with which I was familiar. I cannot recall attending a single lecture. They were offered but a tacit agreement excused the interns. This was not benevolent, but realistic, for whenever we sat down and were not eating we fell asleep. Like the children, it was always past our bedtime.

Much has been written about the difficulties immigrants experience in adapting to a new culture; problems with the language, the diet or their work. I suffered none of these. What I did miss—sport—surprised me but was of no consequence in the first months as I had no spare time. Later, as I became efficient, sometimes a short interval was free and I wanted to escape from the hospital. A tavern on Monument Street opposite the clinic presented a refuge. It had a television, a novelty to me. The set was tuned permanently to the sports channel and I could nurse a small beer while watching. Although it resembled rugby I couldn't understand American football and when I complained that I couldn't see the ball, I was informed, "That's the whole point." The game was accompanied by razzmatazz and interrupted by commercials, which I had never seen. American football resembled American politics: you couldn't and weren't supposed to see the ball until too late.

Baseball, even if I could follow it, lasted for hours and I had only ten minutes. But one sport crossed the Atlantic, instantly recognizable—boxing. Bouts were shown regularly, sponsored by Pabst or Schlitz. Watching boxing gave me a refreshing change from work. One of the attractions of this sport was its brutality, in contrast to my occupation, which was genteel. I was surrounded by women all day and most of the night; listening to them, empathizing with them and imagining myself in their role, the better to envisage their lives. From time to time I needed some contrast. In London, as an antidote to study, rugby had involved pulverizing the opponents or suffering the consequences. Now I had not enough energy to play checkers, let alone rugby. In the tavern I could just lift the cool glass and watch two men doing battle, enjoying the action vicariously.

Dr. Eastman visited the labor floor in the afternoon, taking the only armchair, dilapidated though it was, in the office. He would scrutinize the labor board and discuss any patient, or topic, we raised. For example, determining the weight of a fetus is important because it affects the management of labor and delivery. This estimation was made clinically, by history and palpation. A sweepstakes was held to guess the weights of the newborns, twenty-five cents to enter, winner take all. Dr. Eastman was a formidable competitor, not happy to lose his reputation or his quarter. He questioned the histories and physical examinations in detail.

"How old is the mother?" "How many children does she have and what were the lengths of pregnancy and birth weights?" "Does the mother consider this child will be larger than the others, what is her opinion?" "How much did she weigh at conception and how much does she weigh now?" "How reliable was the menstrual data?" "How advanced is the pregnancy in weeks?" "How tall is she and how tall is the father?" "What is the presentation, vertex, breech or otherwise?" "Is the presenting part floating, dipping or engaged—if so, how low?" Having assimilated this information he would palpate the pregnant abdomen, write his estimate in grams on a slip, and drop it, together with a quarter, in the pot. Subsequently, when the baby was born and weighed, the winner would be posted and enriched.

The problem with this weight estimate was that, like other observations, it was most accurate where it mattered least. In the range between 2500 grams (5 1/2 lbs.) and 4100 grams (9 lbs.) estimates were accurate, but it was easy to err on both ends of the scale and miss a large baby, which may weigh 5500 grams (12 lbs.) in a large mother. Vaginal delivery could be dangerous in such cases. Similarly, accuracy diminished at the low end, a fetus weighing 1600 grams (3 1/2 lbs.) could easily be overestimated in a small mother. Such low birth weight children did not do as well as they do now, particularly if they also suffered infection.

A family atmosphere prevailed among the house staff, for at least half were married and living in the compound with their children. Mothers walked the children and pushed baby buggies through the hospital courtyard in the late afternoons and sometimes it was possible to join them. We singles were invited to supper and it was then that I first read stories to children, which pastime I later enjoyed more than any other task of fatherhood. Sharing this domesticity made my separation easier to bear.

I was one of a trio of friends, the first time I had experienced such a grouping. Dwain, a second-year resident, had been brought up on a farm near a small town in Minnesota, and the only cities he knew were Chicago and Minneapolis, where he had attended college and medical school respectively. He could fix anything mechanical, was informed in the ways of nature, able to identify crops and trees at a glance, and was knowledgeable about animals and their habits. Hunting, which he had learned as a child, was his passion. He was single, a devout Catholic who conducted his life strictly according to their beliefs.

All these traits were lacking in my fellow intern Dey and me. Dey was also single and Catholic but was Dwain's opposite. He wore his religion lightly, yet he was a theologian and formidable in debate, having been schooled by the Jesuits. He could explain the historical basis and evolution of the tenets of the faith but he did so dispassionately, questioning some of them. Dwain first regarded this as heresy, never having been exposed to a dissection of his absolute faith. I was a religious illiterate and a spectator, uninformed, at these debates. The British view was that religion was acceptable in small doses but did not define a person. It was bad form in England to ask anyone what his religion was, worse to announce it, and debating it was quite outside the pale. People were judged by how they behaved, not what they believed.

Dey was European, sophisticated and cosmopolitan, and in addition to impeccable English he spoke Dutch, German, French and Italian. He had worked in the laboratory at Cambridge, studying oxygen pressures in animals. Following this he served two years in the Dutch Air Force as a medical officer in an experimental unit studying the effects of varying oxygen pressures on pilots at high altitude. He was a research physiologist specializing in blood gases who was also an obstetric intern. I do not recall how Dr. Eastman recruited him but he had chosen wisely. Dey was a delightful companion, an excellent talker with a trenchant opinion on a wide variety of issues. But, in the event that I were shipwrecked on a desert island Dwain would have been my choice as a companion, for then I would have had a sporting chance of survival. If Dey and I were stranded we would have died in short order, still talking simultaneously.

Whenever schedules permitted we three took a drive together in Dwain's trusty Chevy. Dey paid for gas while I contributed by washing and polishing the vehicle inside and out as I enjoy cleaning things (floors, furniture, silver, rugs and cars). We parked the car outside the psychiatric wing and one Sunday morning I was lovingly polishing the curving rear fender when a psychiatric resident walked by. "I presume you know that what you are doing is a substitute for intercourse," he remarked, unasked. To say I was taken aback is an understatement. He did not know me or my circumstances of separation, and I thought he must be psychic, well suited to his trade.

We made short trips, anywhere to get away from the hospital—first to Loch Raven, where we strolled beside the Lake, then to Gunpowder Falls, walking along the river bank and listening to the water tumbling over the boulders. Good as the hospital food was, we enjoyed a change and located an inn where we ate beside the log fire or outside overlooking the lake, as the weather dictated. Fall was lovely, the woods transformed. Later, as we had more time, we widened our excursions to Annapolis and other destinations on the Chesapeake Bay. Baltimore blossomed in the spring and we drove north up Charles Street through Homeland, where the daffodils and tulips were followed by dogwood, almond blossoms, azaleas and rhododendron in the gardens of the slate-roofed colonial stone houses. A stream rippled beside the quiet roads, interspersed with pools and fountains.

Dey remained at Hopkins in research and gained an international reputation. Later he moved to Washington, D.C., and joined a foundation, where he wrote and spoke on ethical issues. I noticed a quote in a magazine, "Doctor dissident voice in liberal sex meeting." Asked his opinion on the new mores and sexual promiscuity, the M.D., Ph.D. responded, "'Intercourse without love and commitment is merely genital calisthenics.'" The style and voice were Dey's.

Dr. Eastman's teaching emphasized "Keep it simple." The senior residents who were up to date with the most recent reports and newer procedures asked him why he had not included one of the latter in the latest edition of his textbook. He replied that in small rural hospitals the babies were delivered by general practitioners. A copy of his book was in the delivery room suite but it was only read when the doctor was faced with a complication he might not have encountered previously. In such circumstances, often alone in the middle of the night, the doctor was consulting him by proxy and a clear description of one established method to deal with the complication, rather than a discussion of alternative procedures, was the safest advice to give. When a new method was proven to result in a superior outcome, it was introduced at the expense of its predecessor. The research and testing phases were not included. This explanation was received with skepticism and I suspect that I was the only one of his listeners who, within four years, was practicing in a thirty-bed hospital in a rural area. From this experience I can vouch for the truth of his argument.

He called on us to obey the first rule of medicine—"do no harm"—and warned us about "meddlesome obstetrics," which he detested. A minimum of intervention was needed in a physiological process such as pregnancy and delivery; observation, yes, but interference, no. He was adamantly opposed to "perineal obstetrics," by which he meant that all attention was directed to the doctor being present at the crowning (distention of the perineum by the baby's head), the labor having been neglected. Some doctors resented being called too early and their displeasure was exceeded only by being called too late. The labor nurse had to concentrate her skills on this timing, leaving less for care of the mother and monitoring of the fetus.

In the past, women with chronic disease had been denied motherhood. They may not have lived to reproductive age, or might have been so ill that they failed to ovulate. Those who did conceive frequently had a stillborn baby, for example, diabetic women or those with Rh incompatibility. Medical advances had had a happy byproduct in that many women who had their disease controlled could now become pregnant and deliver a healthy baby. This presented obstetricians with new challenges and the array of medical problems complicating pregnancy widened dramatically. Hopkins received referrals of complicated cases, one of which was a pregnant woman dying of leukemia who had to survive until her fetus reached viability, and then be sectioned. It was not an acute situation, such as a postmortem abdominal delivery immediately after a traffic fatality, resulting in a living baby, which I had seen in London, but it was challenging. This death was slow and the nurses and interns came to know the patient, sitting beside her, holding her hand as life ebbed. It sounds a melancholy task yet it was not—the reverse, in fact, as her determination to live shone through and life continued in her child.

Obstetrics is unique in that two lives are linked and consequently ethical dilemmas arise, which are now discussed by committees composed of ethicists, lawyers, ministers, nurses, psychologists, doctors, and other disciplines as appropriate. This is an improvement over what prevailed when I was in practice, when all decisions were made by the doctor in charge. In 1953, ethical problems were fewer and simpler. Dr. Eastman taught a single creed: "Death is the enemy."

I was driving on an expired British license, which might have precipitated another minor statutory problem besides the ones Dr. Eastman had mentioned earlier in his letter. One day I unexpectedly had an hour free, so left the hospital in my white uniform and caught the bus downtown to the examining office to apply for a Maryland license. I left the Chevrolet safe in our street parking spot. Managing to pass the written test I lined up for the driving section. My examiner inquired "O.K., doc, where's your car?"

"I don't have a car," I replied.

"You're the only doc I ever met without a car. How'd you get here?"

"By bus," I said, "and I have to get back to Hopkins Women's Clinic before they miss me." "Then the State will give you a lift," he volunteered, "get in my car and drive us back to the hospital." I thanked him and started cautiously, waiting inordinately long before crossing the stream of traffic and waving my arm out of the window to indicate a turn.

"Doc," he said, "please stop all that nonsense, just drive. I want to ask you a question." He then confided in me, saying that his wife had been ill for some months with irregular vaginal bleeding, particularly on contact. She had seen two doctors, each of whom had made a different diagnosis, one prescribing pills, the other a suppository. Neither had taken a cervical smear or biopsy. We had now reached the hospital and he asked where I entered. "By the back door on Wolfe," I replied. "We need to park for a few minutes."

"Pull up by that fire plug," he instructed, pointing to the only vacant space in the block. I ascertained that his wife was still bleeding and he said that she was sicker and getting weak. She had had to stop work and he was short of money and faith in doctors. The history and symptoms suggested cervical cancer, and I explained that this possibility must be investigated soon and treatment begun. "Write down her name and address, wait here and I'll get her seen by a good doctor," I said, then went to the gyn cancer clinic, made the arrangements, and brought him the appointment and some encouraging words.

"Thank you, doctor, very much," he replied. "By the way, you made a perfect score on the test, whad'ya know. I'll have them mail you your driving license." This was my first fee-for-service case in America.

I was by now indoctrinated in the Hopkins method of taking and recording an obstetric history. The litany of questions, in a predestined order with no free form allowed, would have driven a psychiatrist crazy. The way we collected facts was methodical, systematic, complete, but it still had style. The completed history was best heard as a recitation rather than seen as a record. It could not be confused with any other presentation, being unique. Although others ridiculed our apparent compulsiveness, the variations in sequence and outcome of pregnancy are considerable and require adequate cataloging. Our records enabled Dr. Eastman to gather many details concerning pregnancy, labor, and delivery for each patient we served. He invited me to his office one day and showed me his sorting machine, which stood in an adjacent corridor—the tool he used to analyze this data. Each patient's chart was abstracted and eighty facts were punched into the numbered slots on a rectangular card. The cards were then entered into the machine, which was programmed to select those with certain numbered slots punched. When switched on, the machine shot out the required cards into a receptacle, accompanied by a fluttering noise resembling a flock of birds settling in a tree. Watching his demonstration I understood how he obtained the numbers for his book and lectures. From the thousands of cards, each representing a baby delivered, he first selected those who suffered from premature rupture of the membranes. The machine indicated the total numbers of cards processed and the number selected, which provided a percentage. Then, using the sample, you could choose subgroups by age, parity, duration of pregnancy and complications such as infection. In each instance you knew the outcome for the baby as this was included in the eighty facts recorded. This all depended on the accurate recording that we supplied, using the Hopkins obstetric history.

"Yes, you were correct, Dick," he told me, smiling (during nine years of training, he was the only chief who called me Dick), "obstetrics does lend itself to enumeration." He was repeating the observation I had made in my letter of application, in which I had stated that it occurred to me after hearing his lecture. I had suspected it was this comment that had motivated him to employ me, and now he confirmed it. Ironically, circumstances prevented me from working under him in research using this method.

Unexpectedly, my fellow intern Mark invited Dey and me to accompany him and his wife Martha, and their young son, to Atlanta for Christmas. Regretfully, we explained that we were working, only to find that the schedules had been skillfully juggled by the U.S. half of our team. (Americans are masters of logistics because they start with the assumption that anything is possible.)

We left in the early evening, and drove through the night, travelling 700 miles in fourteen hours. Dey and I had never experienced a car trip of this duration and we reveled in the novelty, freedom and adventure. We first passed through Washington, which we knew as Dwain had taken us there. We drove south to Richmond, then west to Greensboro, Charlotte and Atlanta. At that time there were no interstates, so we passed through small towns in Virginia and the Carolinas on rural routes. The houses, churches, stores and some of the barns were decorated with Christmas lights, lavish to my eye accustomed to the frugality of England. The farther we travelled, the warmer it became, almost balmy, and the night scents of the South were on the air. It was a magical trip and it concluded when Mark's parents greeted us in the morning. Their house was large, with a guest house adjoining, all standing in a compound of some acreage with boundaries marked by a white picket fence. Their hospitality was lavish and we relaxed in sumptuous surroundings. I had forgotten what leisure was, being able to sleep with never a care for the morn, dress in wool instead of a stiff uniform and with no telephone to summon me, just a gentle invitation to a meal or chat. Flowers in crystal vases, camellias in bloom, bourbon in decanters, a piano played softly, formed the backdrop. Our hosts conveyed the feeling that it was a privilege to have us share their family, home and Christmas. The hours passed swiftly and soon we headed North. I was unable to thank Mark and his parents adequately for making my first Christmas in America so memorable.

The change to gynecology was welcome and the schedule remained the same; two months were to be spent in the clinics, emergency and operating rooms, one month each at a time. I was looking forward to the OR, one month of which was on the private service where the majority of cases were those of the chief, Dr. Richard TeLinde. He and Dr. Eastman were dissimilar, except that both were workaholics and the sole authors of the standard textbooks in their respective fields. Dr. Eastman's strengths lay in his global approach to obstetrics and his vision of the future. Dr. TeLinde, in addition to being an excellent surgeon, a succinct and prolific author, was a gynecologic pathologist. He was the only surgeon under whom I studied who had such an interest in gross and microscopic pathology. He conducted a busy private practice, seeing patients every afternoon. In forty years I did not encounter another surgical chief of an academic department with a practice approaching his in numbers of patients or procedures. He was reputed to earn in excess of two million dollars annually. In 1953 this was, as Rolls used to say of the power of their engines, adequate.

It was the duty of the intern to meet Dr. TeLinde at 6:30 AM daily. He drove an old Plymouth, which I presume he parked on the street, for no one would steal it. He displayed none of the ceremony to which I had become accustomed at the Middlesex. He had a limp but walked so quickly down the long corridor to the private wing at the front of the hospital that I had to hurry to keep in step. He was laconic, wasting no time in small talk, asking terse questions concerning the condition of the post-op patients he was to visit. Accompanied by the staff nurse and intern he made quick rounds, issued clear orders and missed nothing. Then our steps were retraced down the corridor and he questioned me about the surgical list for that day—the procedures, the pathology, the patients and any complications. Before 7:30 AM the first incision was made and, like many surgeons, he relaxed and began to talk, usually teaching. Sometimes he described the history of the procedure, who had pioneered this approach, what refinements had been added, and how the results had improved over time. I enjoyed this, for I had not met a surgeon before with such a sense of history of the craft. By mid-morning his secretary appeared, suitably garbed, and went through the mail. He dictated concise replies and dealt with the day's correspondence and messages (while continuing to operate). I had experienced this before in Wales, but apparently it was unusual in an American surgeon and I never again witnessed this routine. Lunch, a welcome interlude, was taken early. We ate in a small crowded back room communally with the nurses, feasting on delicious sandwiches from a nearby market. To save time we did not remove our surgical gloves, merely washing them before eating. This meant that when we returned for the next case they were stripped off and we had only to do a short scrub, easier on the hands. Some did not relish eating with gloves on but I had no such compunction.

Dr. TeLinde increased his surgical output by using two adjacent rooms, a major in one followed by a minor in a smaller room, giving time for the major room to be readied again—an efficient method which I subsequently copied. Surgery, except for emergencies was over by 2:00 PM, when he started seeing private patients in his office downstairs. A time/motion expert should have studied him.

When visiting one of Dr. TeLinde's post-op patients on evening rounds I found the room in darkness but for a bedside light, and as I approached I could see something first glowing on the bedclothes and then waving in the air, sparkling. I finally realized it was a solitaire diamond, the largest I had seen. A year before this, during my final oral examination, one of my examiners in ob/gyn had been a woman wearing a diamond ring with a large stone. I had admired her for gaining prominence in our discipline, as women were a rarity in 1953. I had imagined she had earned the money to purchase this fine ring, thoughts that had distracted me from the questions she posed. But the diamond I now saw was in a different league and its owner did not question me, but said in a southern drawl, "Honey, come sit by me. I'm fine but you look tired and sad."

I sat on the bed (unprofessionally) and admitted being tired. Under her sympathetic prompting I told her my story and she responded, "That's terrible, being parted from your bride for so long, but she's a doctor and coming over to join you, that's romantic." Then she invited me to bring

Kate to her home in Montgomery, Alabama, for a vacation any time at all. They had a guest house on their property and Clyde would be delighted to have us visit, she assured me, and she gave me her card.

Late that night I had a call, waking me from precious sleep. An indignant nurse bleated, "There's a man in one of Dr. TeLinde's patient's rooms and that is not permitted. You must come and evict him."

"Who is the patient?" She named my friend of the giant solitaire.

"This is not a medical matter, it falls under the purview of nursing."

"Oh no it doesn't. Will you do something or shall I wake Dr. TeLinde?"

"Please don't be hasty, what is the man doing?"

"He's wearing a silk dressing gown, sitting on her bed and smoking a large cigar, which is also forbidden."

"Well, while he's smoking the cigar no damage is likely to occur to our patient. Please check and see if the patient's husband has been admitted."

(Pause.) "Yes, he has, for cardiac screening, and there's nothing wrong with him."

"Good, it is a connubial visit, beneficial to both parties. I suggest we wait for thirty minutes. I predict it will be self-solving so do not let us disturb or inform Dr. TeLinde," I replied, and promptly fell asleep.

Half an hour later the phone woke me again. "I hate to admit it but you were right," said the nurse. "He's left and given us a large box of chocolates."

My time with Dr. TeLinde was limited and I wanted to ingratiate myself with him. I thought he must have some relaxation—surely he couldn't work like this fifty-two weeks a year (or could he?). Someone told me that Dr. TeLinde permitted himself one extravagance—salmon fishing in Canada—and that he was in fact flying there on the coming weekend. Spurred by this I visited the library to study this arcane pursuit, as all I knew of salmon was that I preferred the fillets to the steaks and poached to grilled. I attempted to grasp the lore of the sport and ascertained the names of some Scottish salmon rivers.

The next Monday morning, when we were scrubbed, I decided to make my cast, and inquired if Dr. TeLinde had spent a pleasant weekend—the first personal remark I had ever ventured. He replied that he had been salmon fishing in Canada and, under gentle prodding, described his trip. I asked if he had fished in Scotland, to which he replied sadly that he never had the time. Reassured by this, I expatiated on the River Dee near Balmoral, the Queen's castle in the Scottish Highlands. (Here I was skating on thin ice, for like any Londoner I knew little of Scotland. But I felt the discussion went well and that we two would be bonded forever by salmon.) This was my last week in his service, so on the following Saturday at noon I visited his office, seeking some form of recommendation—a letter, a promise, anything would do. Alas, I had misjudged the man. He was in no mood to talk to me about salmon or anything else. Desperate, I persisted, accompanying him across the road to the barber shop. It was difficult to talk above, over, and around the barber, and to convey my sentiments and predicament in public. I told him I felt privileged to have been taught by him and that I was leaving shortly. Could I please have his signature on some article that would demonstrate I had served him? I had in mind an autographed copy of his textbook. He responded grudgingly that I should run back to his office, ask his secretary for a small photograph of him, and return. This I did and he signed it after enquiring my name and how to spell it. My fishy ruse had, deservedly, availed me nothing and I felt rejected.

The year ended with a revue given by the students and house staff for the faculty, on a hot and humid evening in a crowded hall. This evening was reminiscent of the Christmas concert party at the Middlesex but the humor was less benign.

The faculty sat in front and were served mint juleps. House staff were seated in the middle and students at the back; both drank beer. The famous entered singly and the young serenaded them with vigor. The pathologist, a Dr. Pitsch, came in—"Pitsch, Pitsch you son of a bitch," sang the students. Dr. TeLinde took his place: "Show us your two million dollar fingers," they shouted. He waved two digits of his right hand.

The opening skit was dated June 30, 1953. A tall, robust, handsome young man, elegantly dressed, entered, burdened with sports equipment—golf clubs, skis, tennis racquet, scuba gear, ice skates and fishing rods. An older man greeted him obsequiously, fawning, "Welcome to Hopkins, doctor." Curtain: new date, June 30, 1954. The tallest, thinnest man we had shuffled in, stooped, naked but for a loin cloth. He appeared jaundiced, as he was painted yellow. He paused, then coughing violently, he spat large clots of blood into a tin cup, all he possessed. The greeter from the previous skit reappeared, dominant, hostile and threatening, and he snarled, "Get out."

This was topical. An intern, scion of a Boston surgical family from Harvard, had been one of my two roommates. He had become ill with fever, coughing bloody sputum, accompanied by weakness and weight loss, but had continued to work until he could no longer climb the six flights to our room. Finally, after numerous investigations and incorrect diagnoses, by surgery, the medical service had found the answer to be a rare infection and he had been returned to Boston for treatment and convalescence.

Medical dynasties were common at Hopkins, and in addition to my unfortunate roommate there were three men on the faculty who were sons of distinguished fathers, but whose lustre did not match that of their forebears. A trio sang a ditty, the refrain of which ran along these lines: "We are three sons of our daddies, three chips off the old block." Each had a verse more cruel than the last. The subjects of this derision managed to smile, with, I surmised, considerable effort.

As time passed the room grew hotter, more liquor and beer were drunk, and the audience became raucous. A skit followed, depicting a small group of the elite preparing for a card game. These men had been studied closely, every mannerism noted, and there was little chance that their fellow audience members would not identify them. One physician, prominent internationally and proud of it, was renowned as a tightwad. A surgeon, known as a gambler and braggart, suggested high stakes. The former wrung his hands in alarm and cried, "I'll stake my reputation." "We don't play for peanuts," came the terse reply.

I did not realize then but do now why the jokes had a bitter taste, beyond satire, verging on the vindictive. First, there was the intensity of competition that pervaded Hopkins at the student, house staff, and faculty levels. The institution attracted ambitious, striving types, rewarded elitism, and eschewed mediocrity. Competition was keener in the U.S. than in England—I had approved of that and had taken a calculated risk in entering the fray. The second thing that distinguished this entertainment from the mellower Middlesex revue was that the Hopkins artists and audience were exclusively male. In contrast, the London show included all members of the Middlesex family, which meant that women predominated.

Hopkins was organized according to a "pyramid system"—which was responsible for some of the competitive atmosphere. In a four-year program we had only three obstetrics residents, one each for years two, three and four, but six interns for the first year. Gynecology had the same. It was obvious that only one of us could advance to the second year and eventually complete the four years. The remaining five would have to go elsewhere to complete their training. No one in our group had talked about this, and in fact there was no competition in our small circle, for we six had collaborated, supported, and covered one another in order to survive the year.

My letter of invitation had stated "to serve an internship." No mention had been made of a residency, but it was nonetheless June before I realized that only one person could remain, and I knew it would not be me as I was not the best qualified. I did not have the best intellect; Maurice from Harvard held that distinction. Dey was pre-eminent in research capability, Steve from Memphis was the most resilient and optimistic, and José and I were equal in clinical experience. Mark from Princeton was poised, with the best temperament and equanimity, allied to a sound theoretical and practical knowledge.

My intuition was promptly confirmed. Dr. Eastman summoned me and explained that he regretted there was not room to keep all those who merited it. He would arrange for me to go to any hospital I chose for the remaining three years. I had no idea what to do or say. Sensing this, he recommended either Los Angeles County Hospital, to serve under my namesake, Dr. Daniel Morton, or Kings County Hospital in Brooklyn, another large service. I then told him, for the first time, that I had no money and a wife who would graduate in October and hoped to be a pediatrician. Learning this, he responded that he had more influence in New York, where the chief, recently appointed, was a former member of his faculty. He promised to call and see what could be arranged.

The next day he informed me that if I went to Brooklyn, Kate could join the pediatric program in October and that residential accommodation was available for us in the hospital at no charge. Our salaries would be seventy-five and fifty dollars per month and neither program was pyramidal. I thanked him, accepted, and he gave me a large signed portrait and wished me well. That was the last time I saw Dr. Eastman.

There is a law of diminishing returns in training (learning is not proportional to the time spent). In this first year I learned, not twenty-five percent, but over sixty percent of what I eventually knew clinically in all three domains of learning: facts (head), skills (hands), and attitude (heart). In the next two years, thirty percent was added as my experience, especially in obstetrical complications, increased. The fourth year added the remainder—surgical techniques, which can only be taught one-on-one. But the Hopkins year left an indelible mark for which I remain grateful.

In deciding to go to Kings County I had had, unfortunately, to ignore a military maxim in which I believed: "Time spent in reconnaissance is never wasted." I had no time or money to visit Brooklyn, Los Angeles, or other university hospitals.

Chapter 5

In the Shadow of Ebetts Field

Leaving Hopkins, I rode the bus back to New York, burdened with two suitcases. Then I braved the subway bound for Nostrand Avenue, Brooklyn. A veteran of the London Underground, I found the New York version confusing, dirty, and primitive. It was rush hour, hot and humid. Arriving at Times Square, I inquired "How, please, may I reach Brooklyn?"

"Take the Brooklyn train."

"How, please, may I reach Kings County Hospital?"

"My mother died there."

This type of exchange continued but I finally reached my goal and trudged through the trash-filled streets to the hospital.

The size of the complex was daunting, for it covered several blocks along Clarkson from New York Avenue in the west to Utica Avenue in the east. The majority of the buildings were old, but new construction was underway for a medical school. The delivery rooms were on the eighth floor of the main hospital block, and I reached them in the evening still carrying my suitcases, hot, tired, hungry, thirsty and dispirited.

A few other newcomers had arrived and a meeting was convened by a senior resident. He asked about our history and experience and told me I was on duty for the delivery rooms, supervising the interns and students and reporting to him. The schedule was the same as at Hopkins.

The hospital had 1,200 beds in the main structure and more in separate buildings dotting the campus. A tuberculosis unit filled one building, an acute psychiatric unit another, and chronic cases were in the adjoining state hospital. There were isolation units, one filled with poliomyelitis patients and one with prisoners, largely from Sing Sing. Fifteen thousand babies were delivered a year (forty-one daily), compared with 3,600 at Hopkins. The patients were similar to those at Hopkins in that they were all poor, but the ethnic proportions differed. In Baltimore over ninety-five percent of our patients were black, whereas in Brooklyn only fifty percent were, thirty-five percent being Puerto Rican and fifteen percent white.

I was confronted by over four times as many deliveries every day as I had known. The rate of complications was higher and the supervision lower, with a consequent increase in responsibility. This was welcome, but I was depressed at leaving Hopkins, and needed my own project to find solace. What could I turn to that would be absorbing? Research seemed the answer, although I knew little about it. Research means the acquisition of new knowledge, but one needs to know first what is unknown in order to advance the borders of the subject. Thus, within a week of having left him, I called Dr. Eastman and asked him to suggest a simple research project.

Surprised, he inquired what resources I had in my new situation. I answered, "none," explaining that I was on the delivery floor for six months, during which time 7,500 babies would be born. He promised to ruminate on this and called the next day, saying that it was unknown how frequently proteinuria (protein in the urine, considered abnormal) occurred during labor in a healthy woman. Labor is well named, for it is hard work—exercise, in fact—and it was known that proteinuria occurred in athletes of both sexes following competition. However, in pregnancy proteinuria has a special significance as it is one of the three signs of toxemia. Therefore, it was important to distinguish between the appearance of protein in the urine due to toxemia, an abnormal condition and proteinuria as a normal response to the exercise of labor. He recommended that I consult a friend of his, Dr. Leon Chesley, an expert on toxemia, and gave me his number. When I called I was surprised to learn that Chesley worked in the same hospital as I did. He was a scientist who had studied toxemia experimentally throughout his career and had published many articles and books on the topic. He was charming, overlooking my ignorance and inexperience. Without his help the project would not have been started, completed, or published. Fortunately, there was a simple test for proteinuria which I could perform in the delivery floor lab. We studied over 600 mothers and demonstrated that proteinuria occurred frequently in healthy women in labor. By examining the histories of our patients we identified three factors that made the condition more likely in some women than in others, and constructed a simple table to display this. Due to the eminence of my partner, who insisted I be first author, our paper was published in 1956.

Later Dr. Eastman sent me an autographed copy of the new edition of his textbook with a reference to the page on which our table was reproduced.

From the house staff dormitory in which I shared a small room—the only size they had—I could see the top of a large building, the function of which puzzled me. I asked my roommate what it was and his reply, "Ebetts Field," did not enlighten me. I must have been the only resident of the borough in July 1954 who did not know of the Dodgers and their ballpark, and when my ignorance was revealed a Dodger fan vowed to correct it in order to render me eligible to mix with decent people.

My first visit there was a revelation, for it was a night game and I had never seen sport before under lights. Watching infield practice, I was amazed by the pace of the ball and accuracy of the throws. My tutor spoke the names of the team with reverence—Snider, Reese, Hodges, Robinson, Furillo, Newcombe, Campanella—the litany continued. I marvelled at the colors, the spectators' shirts, the advertisements, the intensity and directness of the comments ("Down his throat, Newk!"). We sat in democratic companionship, quaffing beer, cheering our heroes. The contrast with cricket was striking. Colors there were white for the players, green for the grass. The languid spectators sipped tea, and occasionally some subdued clapping was heard, the opponents given credit as well as the home team.

I remain a novice in baseball, having attended only that first season, but I had the distinction of being taken for Duke Snider. The mistake occurred on the steps leading from the ticket office when, dressed in my whites, I ran down them. A knot of small boys were lingering and one shouted, "Look, there's Snider." "No, he ain't the Duke," snorted his senior. Once, when I was making evening rounds, I was compared to another team member. Following a normal delivery, patients had one day's rest. They were in a large ward and one lady was evidently their leader. When I appeared, her sidekick observed, "Hey, here's a new doctor. He looks like Jackie Robinson." The leader scrutinized me carefully. "Let's just say he's got an arse like Jackie Robinson," she pronounced disparagingly. This was a backhanded compliment, I realized, being by now familiar with her hero's silhouette.

One day a resident approached me furtively. "Would you like to come to the ballgame tonight?"

"Sure, I'm off."

"The Cards are playing," he said conspiratorially, "and I'm from St. Louis."

The significance of these two facts was lost on me; then, arriving at the park he sounded me out. "You're another rabid Dodger fan, I presume?" he inquired.

"Not exactly, I know their names and am trying to learn the game."

Emboldened, he replied, "You'll never learn it from those bums. I'll show you someone who knows how to play the game. Stan the Man Musial." He recited the statistics of his hero, and tried to teach me the subtleties of hitting. When Stan struck, my tutor explained why he had chosen that particular direction, selected that shot: in order to pierce the defense and frustrate the opposition. He was a cerebral player.

Abortion was illegal and the penalties, both criminal and civil, were severe. But demand existed and abortionists flourished. I had had experience of the trade in London and more extensively in Baltimore, where we treated ill women who had undergone criminal abortion, but this had not prepared me for the scope and severity of the problem in Kings County Hospital. Of the 22,000 obstetric patients admitted annually, 7,000 were victims of criminal abortion. We were the hospital of last resort for the borough and treated everyone. We never refused admission when it was indicated and never referred a patient to another facility.

I did not inquire of the circumstances or of the perpetrators of the abortions, for that was not my job. The social service and criminal justice staff would interrogate some of our patients and the relatives of those who died. The mortality rate for our incomplete abortion patients far exceeded that for our deliveries. To have a baby was safer than to abort one. I was told that most of the abortions were performed in New Jersey and the women then traveled back to their homes in Brooklyn. Clearly, many abortions were also performed in Brooklyn and elsewhere in New York City.

Our patients with incomplete abortions were among the sickest I ever encountered. The term "incomplete" refers to the fact that the uterus is not completely empty of the embryo and the placenta. In the typical situation a portion of the placenta is retained, following destruction and expulsion of the embryo. The retained products become infected, and this, coupled with the bleeding from the abortion procedure, creates a serious situation. Young women can tolerate considerable blood loss, and replacement with intravenous fluids, not necessarily blood, will save their lives. But if the anemia is complicated by infection the patient deteriorates rapidly. The infection spreads quickly and widely as the open bleeding vessels in the uterus provide an entry for bacteria. These multiply and are carried by the bloodstream into the muscle of the uterus and then beyond, resulting in infection throughout the body. The bacteria involved are virulent and, having gained hold, overwhelm some organs of the body such as the kidneys, heart and brain.

Treatment was threefold; first, to identify the type of bacteria and flood the blood and tissues with an appropriate antibiotic; second, to treat the anemia with blood or packed red cells; and third, to evacuate surgically the uterus of the infected retained tissue, which was harboring and reinforcing the bacterial invasion. Sometimes it was necessary to remove the uterus, tubes, and ovaries if all were heavily infected, and timing the surgical procedures in conjunction with the medical treatment of infection called for experience and judgment.

The majority of our patients were young, many under twenty, but some were in their late thirties. With mild and moderate cases we moved quickly to empty the uterus by D&C and that, coupled with IV antibiotics, was usually sufficient. We performed the D&Cs starting at 7:00 PM, using two adjacent operating rooms, sometimes doing twenty cases in an evening. They were tricky, for the uterus was soft and it was easy to rupture it with the curette or other instrument. The severe cases who had generalized infection upon admission taught me some medicine, for we then consulted the infectious disease service and learned about different strains of bacteria and how to treat them.

Upon discharge, our patients were all given an appointment at the family planning clinic. But few kept the appointment and we did not have the resources to follow up the no-shows. It is ironic that we treated our patients competently and vigorously, often saving their lives, but did little to prevent recurrence.

The eighth floor was an inconvenient location for the delivery rooms, particularly in emergencies. One afternoon the elevator disgorged a wedding party, gaily attired but somewhat the worse for drink. Our patient was clearly the bride, who had timed matters well. She had used her bridal carriage to convey her and her bemused husband directly from the altar to the delivery table. Her progress was now hindered by her headdress, which had slipped over one eye, impairing her vision. Clutching a bouquet in one hand she steered her smaller husband with the other, shouting simultaneously at her mother. The wedding guests, in varying stages of inebriation, pushed into the labor room gabbling excitedly in Italian.

The nurses, hurrying to get her to the delivery room before it was too late, became embroiled with the clerk, who needed to write down her particulars and attach a wristband for identification. (This was important, for it was possible to confuse the identities of the babies, particularly if several were born in one hour.) The patient was unaccustomed to her married name and had difficulty spelling it in between strong contractions. We finally got her on to a stretcher, and observing her, now horizontal, I became concerned that the baby had partially delivered under the wedding dress and was suffocating. I pushed into the fray and asked the nurses to raise her garments. I knew little of women's attire, being accustomed to seeing them fully dressed or naked. The nurses raised layer after layer of clothing, exclaiming over the material, identifying and commenting on every fabric as if it were a fashion show. Finally we could see the perineum, fully distended, and the patient, relieved of her burden of satin, chiffon and silk, gave a triumphant push and delivered a large baby, who immediately cried loudly, adding to the hubbub. The new mother, now responsible for two entries in the borough records within an hour, screamed the joyous news to the baby's grandmother, who, wisely, had been excluded from the accouchement.

Now that all was well I felt the need for a breath of fresh air and some solitude and rode down to seek it. On reaching the ground the elevator operator stopped the elevator about an inch above the floor and opened the gate. Before I could leave, a latecomer from the wedding party pushed forward into the elevator and fell full length. "Why the hell can't you run this thing right?" he shouted at the operator.

"Why the hell can't you look where you're going?" responded that worthy.

Staggering to his feet, the visitor dispensed with talk and hit our employee with a left jab, whereupon our man moved inside and countered with a right hook and they spilled out of the elevator into the lobby. Spectators quickly gathered, formed a ring and shouted encouragement, and the bout looked promising, a three-round amateur warmup. Unfortunately, there wasn't time to organize any betting before the hospital policeman arrived, a beefy experienced veteran. He watched for a couple of minutes, hoping a knockout would simplify his task, but discovering they were well matched and a split decision was likely, he entered the ring during a clinch and shouted "break, break" like a referee.

Grasping the two breathless fighters by their shirt fronts, he said to our man loudly, "Oughta be ashamed," then quietly, "You had 'im, Pat," and released him. Now he held the visitor with both hands and pulled him close, eyeball to eyeball, and bellowed, "Get out you bum! And don't you—never—come—back." The recipient of this advice retreated, cursing, into the arms of his supporters, honor satisfied. To the crowd the cop cried, "O.K. folks, break it up, fun's over, visiting time ends at five." To Pat he said, "Well done, you taught him a lesson, now you need a rest. Put up the out-of-service sign, I'll fix it with Mike."

In mid-October Kate passed her finals with honors, declined the offer of a house job in medicine at the Middlesex, and sailed for the U.S. aboard the *Île de France*, ending our sixteen-month separation. In anticipation, my emotions swung from exultation to anxiety. I feared that she would be disillusioned with me, Brooklyn, Kings County, our accommodations, and my lack of social life, car and money. We had lost all our supports—England, the Middlesex, our families and friends—all we had left was medicine. How would we become friends, regain intimacy, meeting as strangers in a foreign land?

The long-awaited day arrived. I had borrowed a snazzy convertible from my only affluent acquaintance, so I put the top down to make the best of matters. Arriving in Manhattan I got lost in Chinatown. On reaching the river I could see the ship already moored, so I was late. Wearing my hospital whites and using a car with M.D. plates, I bluffed my way past the guard and onto the dock, claiming that I was meeting a handicapped patient who needed immediate transportation to the hospital. It was true, for Kate was handicapped—stuck with me—and had no place to go but the hospital.

I parked perilously close to the water and spotted her, laughing in the center of a group of young people. Her blond hair shone in the morning sun. She appeared taller than I remembered, and younger. I felt overcome, scarcely able to believe she was mine. I jumped from the car, advancing toward her with a sappy look on my face, grinning like a Labrador. On reaching her I realized she did not recognize me.

This was not surprising, as my once-curly locks had been cut. My ballast had shifted south so I resembled a bowling pin rather than the inverted triangle I had been. My whites completed the disguise.

Eventually realizing the awful truth, she greeted me. "Richard dear [never Dick], let me introduce you. Here are Peter, John, and Alice."

"We must leave," I said rudely, "I'm double-parked." Gone were all the romantic declamations I had rehearsed.

The tension between us was dispersed as I promptly got lost again and Kate took the map, asking for our destination. I had a romantic idea, a rare occurrence. "To the Queens Midtown Tunnel, please." We would drive south on the BQE and enjoy the view of the Manhattan spires glinting in the sun, then stop in a park by the ocean before we faced the hospital.

Once we were engaged in a task as partners, Kate directing while I drove, it was as if we had never been apart. When an hour had passed I turned reluctantly up Rockaway to Linden and the Hospital, our home-to-be for two years.

As ten days intervened before Kate had to start work, I requested "passionate leave," which was granted. Where should we go for a second honeymoon that would introduce her to her new country, and do so economically? We had a friend in need, warmhearted and rich, my patient of the solitaire. So, without calling, and hoping it would be romantic to surprise our hosts, we embarked on a 1,000-mile journey to Montgomery, Alabama. (A friend lent us his beat-up VW Beetle.)

When we requested the locals to outline the best route we were told, "If Brooklyn were Venice, Flatbush would be the Grand Canal. You must leave by Flatbush Avenue, cross the Manhattan Bridge, then take the Holland Tunnel." They had neither interest nor ideas about the remaining [outside New York] portion of the route, about 990 miles. (Their directions reminded me of the Boston dowager who decided to take a road trip to

California, and when her chauffeur asked which route she preferred, said, "James, don't quibble, go by way of Worcester.")

Going west, we followed the 22 to Pennsylvania through the Delaware Water Gap beside the Appalachian Trail, across the Susquehanna to what is now 81, through Maryland and West Virginia into the Shenandoah Valley and the Blue Ridge Mountain Parkway. This territory was perfect in the fall. After England, road travel in the U.S. was a revelation. It was pleasurable and efficient, the country adapted to it. There were motels, primitive by today's standards yet convenient compared to English accommodations (or lack thereof). Kate map-read during the first hours then we alternated driving and I slept, a feat in the VW. (Although an optimist to the last, I confessed to some misgivings over our vehicle, but these proved to be unworthy as the car behaved splendidly.)

We reached Tennessee bound for Chattanooga but got lost in the Great Smoky Mountains. This was disturbing, as ours appeared to be the only VW in the state and it attracted some unwanted attention, especially as it had N.Y. M.D. plates. (We felt a little like the New York couple who were touring in West Texas. They were near the Pecos River, southbound, and reached a four-way stop simultaneously with a new Cadillac and an old pick-up, both bearing Texas plates, facing one another east and west. The New Yorkers waited, whereupon both the other vehicles moved forward and turned south, the truck crashing into the side of the Caddy and disabling it before disappearing in a cloud of dust towards El Paso. The driver of the Cadillac staggered across to the New Yorkers' car and asked, "Did either of you two bastards happen to notice that gentleman's number?") At one particularly harrowing point in our trip a state patrol car, driven by one of Tennessee's finest wearing reflecting sunglasses, tailgated us, then pulled alongside and subjected us to a steely prolonged glare. I managed to drive steadily, appearing both innocent and confident. Finally, he gunned the cruiser and blasted away, my heart rate returned to normal, and we putt-putted on.

We arrived unscathed at twilight and found the house, a southern mansion with white columns and large lanterns, looking like Tara. There was a party in progress. The driveway and surrounds were filled with cars, the smallest being a Buick. The lights in the house were blazing and I could hear a piano. We hid the VW, summoned our courage, and rang the bell, travel-stained and dressed in jeans. A butler appeared and I announced we were the Doctors Morton from New York, requesting an interview with the lady of the house. With aplomb he ushered us in and discreetly led us into a holding pen out of sight of the guests, who were in evening dress.

Our hostess appeared, greeted us warmly and without apparent surprise, and suggested we might like to wash before joining them at dinner. About twenty people were seated at a long table and she first introduced us to her husband, Clyde, at one end, and second to a tall man, well into his cups, seated at the other, whom she addressed as "Governor." In Alabama we had started at the top, for he was "Kissing" Jim Folsom.

A woman was playing the piano and singing, making it difficult to converse, which proved to be just as well. The remainder of the evening passed in a haze—soufflé for dessert, bourbon and brandy in crystal goblets, southern ladies to whom I was introduced, inaccurately, as the surgeon who had operated on their hostess. The Governor questioned us and grasped that we were pediatrician and obstetrician, of which he approved, and from New York, of which he did not.

At last all the guests left save the Governor, who was staying the night, a wise precaution. We escaped to the guest house, fell into bed exhausted and slept deeply. At 6:00 AM I was roused and informed that the Governor wished to see me.

I found him sitting in the back of his limousine, "Alabama 1," holding a paper cup of bourbon. "Get in, Doc, we're going fishing," he commanded.

I did not wish to prove that I was no angler and managed to decline with a modicum of grace. "O.K., you're hung over and wish to crawl back to bed with your bride," he observed, accurately, "but you two are good doctors in the specialties we need. Leave New York and hang your shingle in Alabama."

"But Governor, we have no license here," I pointed out.

Laughing, he said, "Don't worry, I'll fix that and anything else you need. Any friend of Clyde's is a friend of mine. Think it over, Doc." He then tapped on the partition and the big car drove away.

Our hostess informed us that Clyde was leaving that evening for Miami and she was flying to California the following morning, but we were welcome to remain at their home for as long as we chose. Following dinner that evening Clyde asked me to ride along with him, I presumed to the airport. I agreed, but to my surprise, when I got to the car I found him attired in pajamas, dressing gown and slippers, and our destination was the railroad station. We were met by the stationmaster, who led him to a red carpet, along which he walked smoking a cigar, then he entered his own railroad car attached to the end of the train.

We said goodbye to our hostess in the morning and spent five enjoyable days of luxurious idleness, dining and dancing in the club after a day by the pool or touring the countryside. Then, having partaken of southern hospitality, we had to face the real world again and return to Brooklyn.

I had two new experiences in delivering patients, the first of which occurred when a nurse and I were summoned in the middle of the night to deliver a patient in the tuberculosis building, the staff having lost control of the inmates at night. The majority were young and Hispanic, and Spanish was the only language we heard. The corridors and rooms were poorly lit and patients were flitting about, laughing and playing like children. The scene reminded me of "Hernando's Hideaway" in Pajama Game, an apt association considering what was going on.

We managed to convince one of their leaders that we were benign, did not represent authority, and only wanted to deliver a baby. With secrecy, we were escorted upstairs and, in semi-darkness, delivered the baby under the inquisitive eyes of several spectators.

The second experience was poignant. I was called to the isolation unit, a building in a corner of the campus. Patients were housed there when it was suspected they had an infectious or contagious disease, often of an unknown nature. But in this instance the diagnosis was clear. The whole building was filled with poliomyelitis patients. The woman I delivered was one of them. She was in an iron lung, but her labor appeared normal, and her attitude inspired admiration. Although cursed with this affliction, she was euphoric when her baby was born, despite the limitation she would face as a mother.

The "married quarters," a euphemism, were on the top floor of the dormitory. Our room was small. We had little baggage between us, which was fortunate, but we were large people, so when we were both in the room one had to lie on the bed. If we both stood or, worse, moved, we collided or became entangled, even when doing a simple task such as combing hair or getting dressed.

The showers and toilet were down the hall. The only other married occupants were a pair of psychiatrists, a charming black couple who were pleased to greet us as reinforcements. He and I labeled and tried to isolate a "ladies only" toilet and a shower stall with the same designation, but neither of us had any mechanical aptitude, and soon every latch we affixed was broken by an irate male who thought the door was stuck and kicked it in.

The population was shifting as new doctors came and went, so many were unaware of the female enclave. Our wives solved their problem by being assertive and achieved minimal privacy.

The first time a patient asked me to kill her was on the cancer ward. We cared for terminal patients who had reached the limits of curative treatment, either surgery, radiotherapy, or a combination. They were not discharged, for we were testing new methods of pain relief, using continuous infusions of a combination of drugs. Confronted by dying patients for whom you can do nothing the inclination is to pass them by, not out of neglect or aversion but because they represent defeat. As patients weaken, their horizons narrow. There is no mention of discharge, home, or recovery. They retain interest only in the small events of the ward. Sometimes I sat beside the patients, sometimes held their hands, and I would relate an event in my life or tell a story.

One woman, in middle age, appeared stoical. On a Saturday she grasped my hand and said, "I want to die and I know you will help me. Put something into my drip when you change it." I remained silent and she continued softly, "Not tonight, I like Sunday mornings. I can hear the church bells and read the newspaper. I can't face Monday morning. Do it Sunday night, it's quiet then."

The second incident occurred over a year later during my last days at the hospital. The patient had advanced cancer with bony metastases, which were not only painful but disfiguring. One was on her forehead, a protruding, suppurating mass, and others were on her limbs, the first I had seen. She was emaciated, a bony skeleton, but her heart was strong because she was only twenty. No one visited her and no one cared. The nurses disliked her, for she was uncooperative, ignoring authority, shouting and swearing, sometimes throwing things, and inconsiderate of others. I stopped daily, sat and talked to her, but felt useless, since I could not bridge the gulf that separated us and saw only contempt in her eyes. She did not request, she demanded that I kill her, resentful of being in the dependent position of having to ask me but too weak to do it herself even if she had had the means. She told me it was her life, her decision and her right to die.

I was assisting a surgeon who was starting a difficult procedure on a cancer patient. The preparations were lengthy, during which he became tense and irascible because he knew he was incompetent to perform the planned dissection. He made the initial incision prematurely and roughly and an instrument fell to the floor. Swearing, he seized a metal kidney dish and hurled it across the room. Narrowly missing a nurse, it hit the tiled wall and fell with a clatter. The anesthesiologist was a woman, calm and experienced. In the silence that followed this affront, she said, "We must excuse Dr. Smith, for the male menopause is more severe than the female." This further galled him, for, like all effective insults, it had an element of truth. I had never seen a surgeon throw anything and this has remained my sole experience.

Kate joined a group of women doctors who met in various hospitals in New York City. She visited Columbia Presbyterian and returned to describe a remarkable woman, an anesthesiologist, who had taught her how to intubate a newborn infant. This skill is valuable and difficult to acquire. Newborns sometimes inhale mucous and blood at delivery or are affected by drugs given in labor or by bleeding from the placenta before delivery. These factors depress respiration, which, unless promptly corrected, leads to brain damage and death. To rectify this it is necessary first to insert a thin tube into the baby's windpipe. A small laryngoscope is needed and the tube must be placed correctly or it goes into the stomach, a common error. Premature babies are especially at risk of respiratory depression and it is more difficult to intubate a premie than a full-term infant. Few doctors could do this in 1954. Kate was taught, using stillborn babies and cats, by Dr. Virginia Apgar at Columbia. She gave Kate a set of the small tubes and an infant laryngoscope and, more importantly, the skill to use them.

Dr. Apgar's name has been immortalized by a score she devised to assess the well-being of a newborn at birth. To appreciate her achievement it must be considered in the context of her time. Anesthesiology was a minor specialty, lacking esteem. Within anesthesia, obstetrical cases were at the nadir. Babies can be, and for the most part were, delivered without anesthesia. From this lowly position, Dr. Apgar, a woman in obstetric anesthesia, used the fundamental art of medicine—observation—and brought a spotlight to bear on the newborn baby.

In the past, doctors paid scant attention to the newborn. They divided them into living or dead, pronounced their gender and recorded their weight. Apart from these few stark facts, little was noted. Consequently, babies might remain untreated during the first vital minutes of life. Dr. Apgar changed that forever. She devised a method of scoring, using five cardinal signs—heart rate, respiration, muscle tone, reflex irritability and color—to assess, within sixty seconds after birth, the health of the newborn infant and the need for life-saving assistance.

	Sign	Score		
		0	1	2
A	APPEARANCE (color)	Blue Pale	Body Pink Extremities Blue	Completely Pink
P	PULSE (heart rate)	Absent	Below 100	Over 100
G	GRIMACE (reflex response to stimulation of sole of foot)	No Response	Grimace	Cry
A	ACTIVITY (muscle tone)	Limp	Some Flexion of Extremities	Active Motion
R	RESPIRATION (respiratory effort)	Absent	Slow Irregular	Good Strong Cry

There are three levels for each of the five factors. For the highest, the baby scored 2; for the middle, 1, and for the lowest, zero. Thus the score ranged between a high of 10 to a low of zero. In common with many procedures that have stood the test of time the Apgar score is simple. Once mastered, it is easy to measure and, within limits, to interpret. It is universal, for no equipment is needed, and it can be used in any setting where birth occurs.

The paper describing her score was published at a fortunate time, for the discipline of perinatology (around birth) was evolving. Obstetricians and pediatricians who specialized in the care of high risk pregnancies and babies appeared. In this ferment the value of the score was recognized. It was a light that illuminated the condition of the newborn and reflected back a number that alerted the baby's doctors and nurses. Charts were posted in every delivery room throughout the U.S. and now the world.

I recall that she invited Kate and me to dinner. To my surprise she had a convertible and, as it was a pleasant evening, she put the top down. Her apartment was on the Palisades so we crossed the George Washington Bridge at high speed as she shouted and gesticulated, paying scant attention to driving, anxious that we not miss any of the landmarks up, down or across the river. We crouched down, scared, grasping any handhold. On reading tributes to her we found that none failed to mention that "a drive with Virginia was one you would never forget" and we concurred.

About ten years later we attended an international conference on birth defects in London, convened by the March of Dimes. A reception was held in Westminster for foreign guests and, with Kate preceding me, we climbed an ornate staircase to the reception line. Suddenly Kate was confronted by Dr. Apgar, who, recognizing her, boomed in her distinctive voice, "Hello again, and what have you been doing since we met?"

Taken aback, Kate replied, "I've had five children."

"My, you have been a busy girl," laughed Virginia.

In 1973 I was teaching at the Johns Hopkins School of Public Health. Faced with a small class seated around a table I noticed one woman, older than the others. Something about her was familiar. Directly she spoke I knew she was Dr. Apgar and I addressed her as such, saying that it was a privilege to have her in the group. She did not recognize me but I was saddened by her appearance. Her vitality had diminished, her spirit lessened, her stature was bowed. None of the other students knew she was a pioneer, her name meant nothing. That was the last time I saw her.

For her contribution, Dr. Apgar was honored in 1994 by the U.S. with the issue of a stamp bearing her likeness.

— In the Shadow of Ebetts Field —

Kate knew a family who owned an island off Connecticut reached by a causeway. They invited us for a weekend. Their home was at the center of the island, and the guest house, which we occupied, was isolated at the water's edge. When exploring we found a cottage, outside of which a Rolls Royce was being polished by an upstanding man with a striking beard. A voice in an upper-class English accent could be heard reading slowly as if from a book. We then realized that the source of this was not human but a phonograph record. Spotting us, the man asked, in a voice identical to that emanating from the machine, who we were and what we were doing. We reciprocated by asking him the same questions.

Taken aback, he replied, "I am Commander Whitehead," as if that should have been obvious. Persevering, Kate asked what he did for a living. "I promote Schweppes," he answered, and civilly asked us in for a drink of his product liberally laced with gin. We were innocents, for we never watched television, and so we were ignorant of one of the most successful advertising campaigns in existence. Solely due to the Commander's talents, Schweppes had a large share of the national tonic market. It transpired that he had lived in the U.S. for many years but had preserved his accent, as he had demonstrated while polishing his icon, the Rolls, which was his advertising prop and personal conveyance. He was the first "professional Englishman" we encountered. We were attempting the reverse, to integrate ourselves into our adopted country.

It was winter and snowflakes began falling that Sunday afternoon. We were reluctant to leave but the snow rapidly deepened. Our hosts urged us to stay but we explained that the hospital could not function without us. Sliding off the island in our VW we reached the Merritt Parkway, where American cars were stuck in snow drifts. The VW, with good traction, negotiated the narrow lane that remained open.

At midnight we reached Harlem, proceeding down 5th Avenue as the traffic light marshalled nonexistent cars, glowing alternately green, amber, and red in the dying storm. We had Manhattan to ourselves except for a few skiers and the occasional patrol car. We drove slowly the length of the island, savoring the winter wonderland, ours alone.

As the summer of 1956 approached and with it the culmination of my second year in Brooklyn, I was concerned over my meager experience and skills in surgery compared with obstetrics. Yet Kate was being well taught and needed more time to master her craft.

For me, the hospital was purgatory. Our living conditions were miserable, our schedules appeared always in conflict, and we were both chronically tired. We had little time together, and no relaxation or social life. We decided that we did not wish to practice in New York and I should explore a new region of the country, preferably in the West.

I searched the advertisements for a gyn surgical senior residency, a rare bird, which I located in Sacred Heart Hospital, Spokane, Washington, one of the largest private hospitals west of the Mississippi, with 660 beds. I wrote to Dr. TeLinde, asking for a reference and a telephone call on my behalf, and my application was accepted.

We bought the VW, which had served us well, and I packed it with my few belongings. In the last week of June Kate and I said goodbye again for what we expected to be a year.

CHAPTER 6

YOUNG MAN GOES WEST

Facing a journey of 2,560 miles, I was sad to be parted from Kate, glad to be leaving Brooklyn, and excited over a new job. Kate had had a car radio installed as a gift to keep me awake on the journey. The radio proved a welcome companion in New York, relaying classical music to soothe me. When I left the metropolis, I heard popular American music for the first time. Two of the current hit songs seemed especially apropos. The first was macabre, relating a series of fatal automobile accidents, each introduced by a rending crash followed by the cry, "Transfusion!" This made me cautious and I temporarily forgot the first rule of driving, which is to overtake the vehicle in front. The second song, which filled the airwaves from east to west, warned, "Son, you're going to drive me to drinkin' if you don't stop driving that hot rod Lincoln."

I tootled along north and west. As the miles passed, fewer VWs were evident and my vehicle became a novelty, popular with gas station attendants who wanted to examine the air-cooled rear engine. After putt-putting across the plains of the Midwest, I reached the real West in Wyoming. Here I felt lonely, isolated, and yearned for the city. Entering a diner that also sold newspapers I inquired if they had a copy of the New York Times. This, coupled with my strange vehicle and English accent, provoked a hostile reaction, the implication being that if the Wyoming Weekly or Grizzly Gazette were not good enough I could take my custom elsewhere and quickly. But once I had crossed the mountains and entered Washington my spirits rose.

Spokane sits in a valley running east to west. The Spokane River runs through the city, cascading over a series of waterfalls in the city center. The first thing that struck me was how clean it all was after Baltimore and Brooklyn. Spokane was not only clean, it was safe. You could walk about the city after dark with confidence and strangers would greet you. The city styled itself the Capital of the Inland Empire, which comprised the area east of the Cascades and west to the Idaho mountains. The Canadian border was the northern limit and Oregon the southern. The region was agricultural, with dry wheat farming and some irrigated crops, large stands of timber to the north, and orchards in the valleys. The military, particularly the USAF, had several bases, and the Hanford reactor plant was sited 165 miles southwest. Spokane was a transport center, with the railroad from Seattle to Chicago and major truck routes passing through town.

There was snow skiing in the mountains, fishing and water sports on the lakes and rivers. The climate was continental, with wide swings in temperature from winter to summer, and the air was crisp, dry and clear, smog absent and clouds rare. The region was sparsely populated and predominantly white, with immigrants from Scandinavia, Germany, and the Netherlands, frequently via the Midwest. There were few of the extremes of wealth and poverty I had found in New York. People were independent, little concerned with the federal government and less with foreign affairs. Political concerns were limited to state and, particularly, local matters.

Sacred Heart Hospital stands on a hill to the south of the city center. My impression on entering was that it was the cleanest hospital in which I had ever set foot. The floors gleamed and the fittings sparkled. I was not only astonished, I was afraid of falling over.

I was allotted a pleasant bedroom and met the other house staff, about eight, all white males fresh from medical school and serving a rotating internship prior to becoming practitioners in the state. We shared a dining room and a lounge.

I spent my time on the operating floor, which was large, serving general surgery and the array of subspecialties including gynecology. The hospital was operated by a Catholic order and Sister Peter Claver supervised the OR floor and obstetrical service. She was later deservedly promoted to chief executive. A skilled administrator, she was a warm, friendly person who took an interest in others. Fortunately, I was the first incumbent of the gynecologic surgery residency, which had just been approved, presumably on the basis of the large surgical volume. This meant that I could plan my own program but I reported to the chairman of obstetrics and gynecology, a non-salaried rotating position.

Here I was again fortunate, for the incumbent, who was to become my last surgical teacher, was a charismatic, gifted man. Tall and slim, invariably immaculately dressed, he was graceful as a cat. His eyes were amber and expressionless. He and his partner, fifteen years his junior, practiced together efficiently. Their suite across from the hospital contained only one consulting room, which they both used on alternate days, in place of the customary design where each partner has his own. Their schedule mandated one man all day in the hospital, starting early with gyn surgery. The second commenced deliveries, vaginally or by section, then went to the office and saw patients for the remainder of the day. When surgery ended the hospital partner made gyn and obs rounds and went home. The following day they reversed roles.

They spent little time in conversation together, preferring to work. Their system resulted in a large number of cases and the senior, my boss, was reputed to be the leading earner among all doctors in the state in each of the previous five years.

A nurse anesthetist was employed who cared for their obstetric patients and gave epidural anesthesia for delivery. This is safer for the mother than a general anesthetic, which (rarely) may be associated with vomiting, aspiration, and respiratory arrest. Epidural is safe for the fetus, yet provides excellent pain relief and permits the mother to remain awake, able to enjoy the birth. Epidurals were uncommon in 1956, and this was my first experience of them as a routine. Their rarity was due to the skill required to initiate and maintain them safely.

This formidable trio was not universally admired, and several rivals criticized them. As the junior partner remarked, "There are nine partnerships here delivering babies; one using epidurals and eight criticizing." Nevertheless, the results they achieved for their private patients surpassed any I had seen. I operated as the senior partner's assistant and also assisted in urological and bowel procedures. Sister advised me which surgeon to approach and recommended particular cases. The surgical department was headed by a Mayo man, which resulted in the staff deriving from Mayo, ensuring excellent technical standards.

The hospital delivered 6,000 babies annually, the majority to private patients, and there was a clinic service for welfare patients staffed by interns. I taught the interns how to monitor labor and deliver patients, including forceps and sections—a rewarding task, as I enjoyed teaching and watching their proficiency increase. Another duty was conferring with doctors who called in with obstetrical problems. I learned more than my callers from these exchanges, and they proved a good introduction to what was to become my stock in trade, consultation to doctors faced with patients who had ob/gyn complications.

I worked every morning and most afternoons in the OR and was on call twenty-four hours, yet the demands were light compared to those of the previous three years. The hospitality of the attending physicians was a pleasant surprise, for it was lacking in Brooklyn. (I fared less well socially with the nurses. It has already been established that my knowledge of religion leaves much to be desired. This was exposed when I overheard two nurses discussing their plans. One said, "No, we can't go then, we have the Altar Society meeting." I interjected, "That sounds like a progressive group, what do you plan to alter?" My serious inquiry was treated as a bad joke. I was already of no interest to the nurses as I was married and, worse, to a doctor not a nurse. Now it was clear I was also a heretic, which was not surprising since I was from New York.)

The cardiac surgeon asked me to his cabin in Idaho for the weekend. Immediately we arrived it was announced we were to water ski. His boat was a Chris-Craft of gleaming wood, powered by a big inboard, and it was clear that no time was to be wasted on theory. The children diagnosed I was a duffer and giggled in anticipation. I confessed my weight and shoe size and was issued a huge pair of skis, unfamiliar and unwieldy. When I splashed into the water, gasping with cold, even the Labrador peered anxiously down at me. As I drifted behind the boat I could hear the "bubble bubble" of the big engine, increasing my anxiety, but with a tremendous pull, up I came and, for a glorious moment, felt like a god as I skimmed across the lake. This came to an abrupt watery end but, with patience on the part of my host, I eventually learned to water ski. In the evening as the moon shone on the lake, we barbecued steaks. In the morning I walked the dog through the woods, read to the children, and hoped this was an augury for the quality of life in the Northwest.

Learning surgery from the vaginal approach as opposed to the abdominal is difficult. The anatomy is upside down, access is restricted, and visibility is limited. It is a solo procedure, for your assistant can only retract to enlarge the operating field and keep it dry by suction. You are seated instead of standing, yet a stiff neck often results. My new mentor taught me first the most important consideration: the selection of the patients for a vaginal hysterectomy or other procedure. If you err on this you may face complications in the midst of surgery that could have been avoided by choosing the correct operation in the first place, that is, abdominal rather than vaginal. Having learned the indications and pathology to avoid, I assisted several times and then operated myself, with his instructions and assistance. It takes confidence to teach vaginal procedures, for you can only whisper in your pupil's ear. He or she has to dissect, clamp, and ligate. You are sitting in the back seat while your student is driving in the front seat.

My teacher, in advance of his time, considered what the patient wanted and how she saw the operation. One example was incisions. For many abdominal procedures, including sections, we used the Pfannenstiel, a curved incision just above the pubic hair line in a skin crease. At the time this was uncommon compared to the customary—and scarring—central vertical incision. (Again, he selected the cases wisely, for access is restricted with the Pfannenstiel and if you find pathology beyond your reach you have made an error for which your patient will suffer.) He also made a fuss over skin cleansing before surgery and the closing and bandaging, together with the aftercare. Some scoffed at him for this but it resulted in fewer infections and hematomas and less pain postoperatively—also appreciated by the patient. A satisfied patient is an excellent referral source and the converse is also true. The previous three years of my training had correctly emphasized pathology, diagnosis and treatment, together with recognizing and treating complications. Now I was learning to view the illness, surgery and convalescence through the patient's eyes.

Following delivery my mentor's patients were taught by the nurse to perform exercises recently described and popularized by Dr. Kegel. The perineum softens during pregnancy and is distended by labor and delivery. To restore muscle tone, the mother voluntarily contracts and relaxes the perineal muscles, thus strengthening the pelvic floor. This prevents prolapse and lessens urinary symptoms such as stress incontinence. Post-hysterectomy and menopausal patients were prescribed estrogens, which lessen osteoporosis in addition to their other benefits. Such preventive measures were unusual in those days.

In December I had marvelous news. Kate called and said she was leaving Brooklyn, having obtained a post as senior resident at Seattle's Children's Orthopedic Hospital. She would fly to Spokane after Christmas and visit me before starting her last residency year on January 1, 1957.

Her hospital served the entire Northwest. Patients came from Washington, Alaska, Montana, and Idaho. Many of the children were seriously ill, some with rare conditions, and the fatality rate was high. Once arrived and established, Kate took me on rounds, telling me the children's names, reciting their histories, treatment and prognosis. The atmosphere in a children's hospital is poignant, and the nurses and doctors are under continued psychological pressure. They unavoidably become attached to their patients and mourn the loss of a child in a manner not seen in a general hospital. The term "burn-out" was not then coined but it was later used in neonatal units and children's hospitals.

A colleague asked me to join him at Eastern State Hospital, where he conducted a clinic every two weeks and performed surgery. As an inducement he claimed it would be a new experience, which it was. The large hospital, situated a few miles outside town, was for psychiatric patients, acute and chronic, with buildings spread over a campus. The inmates suffered from the normal range of gynecological pathology plus some kinds that were rarely seen, and a small number of obstetric patients were also cared for and delivered. I did not foresee a peculiarity, which was that no history was obtainable from the majority of the patients, and, worse, some told fanciful or false stories. Many women had been there for years and their original medical records were sparse. Most were referred to the ob gyn clinic by a nurse who accompanied them, having observed something wrong such as increasing girth, decreasing weight, or abnormal bleeding. My guide had become accomplished at untangling the confusing leads and interpreting the physical signs. The nurses taught me about self-mutilation, and described how some of the younger and stronger patients escaped periodically and were captured by a man or several men, then subjected to severe and repeated abuse and acts of depravity.

Some patients did not wish to be examined, compounding a difficult situation. The psychiatric hospital was well-equipped with surgical facilities and we operated there, for convalescent care was better undertaken by nurses experienced with these patients.

I performed a vaginal hysterectomy on a patient who had had a complete uterine prolapse. When I visited her on the first post-operative day, she was nowhere to be found. A search was instituted and she was discovered having a bath, soaping herself all over and washing her hair. Consternation prevailed among the aides, accustomed to long periods of bed rest post op, but I noticed that the patient's perineum had healed rapidly and completely, with no infection. (I had been concerned about that, as she was uncooperative, unable to understand or follow instructions, and had no personal hygiene.) Subsequently, I encouraged all my patients who had vaginal surgery to take a bath postoperatively. They liked it. I believed it assisted healing and did not contravene the first rule of medicine, do no harm.

The hospital meals were tasty, superior to those of Hopkins and Brooklyn since they were prepared for a small number. I enjoyed fish on Fridays but in the spring there was an abrupt change. Fish appeared daily and meat disappeared. I suspected there must be a strike affecting meat supplies but when I voiced my suspicions to my fellow residents, they replied, "It's Lent." When I revealed the problem to my chief, he responded with an invitation to dine with him in a men's club downtown that was immune to the Catholic writ. I accepted, but as I had never entered, let alone eaten, at a mens' club I was uneasy over protocol.

When we were seated and I had studied the large menu my confidence plummeted further, for I did not know how to order with assurance. I was rescued by the waiter, an older black man who kindly volunteered to play Jeeves to my Bertie Wooster and guide me through the menu. Sensing my discomfort, he said, "How may I assist you sir?"

I asked, "What do you suggest for an hors d'oeuvre?"

"To plan a meal sir, I recommend you first select the entree and then the hors d'oeuvre, dessert and beverage to complement it."

Impressed, I responded, "To get started, how do you choose the entree?"

"Consider two factors, sir. First, what do you wish to eat on this particular evening, and second, what is the strength and specialty of the restaurant?"

"I would like to eat meat this evening," I said firmly.

"A sound choice, sir, for meat is the specialty here, as it is in all superior men's clubs."

"Which meat then?"

"You look like a hearty eater, sir, and if you are hungry, as most young men are, steak is the answer. In my opinion, the New York cut, best taken rare." I acquiesced and was then guided through the vegetables and sauces, horseradish or mustard. He then permitted me to choose one of the two hors d'oeuvres he recommended and one of the two desserts. He then asked, "What do you care to drink, sir?"

"I usually drink beer."

"Of course, sir, but tonight you may wish to prepare the palate with a dry sherry, which can follow beer if you are thirsty now. With the steak, a red wine, I recommend a Burgundy."

Following the dessert, the cheese trolley arrived and he really showed his paces. Dinner concluded with a fine Calvados. I am indebted to this talented man and have followed his principles ever since through a lifetime of professional travel and dining out.

As my year's service drew to a close, my teacher turned his attention from surgery and patient care to personal advice. "Lose weight and then visit a good tailor," he instructed me with asperity. "Get a decent haircut and pay attention to grooming," he advised brusquely while studying his manicured nails in the light reflected from his gold watch. "Buy an American car and keep it clean," he directed as we glided past my dirty VW in his gleaming Cadillac.

He offered me a job as an associate in their practice at a salary of $700 a month. This was seductive, because I admired the standard of medicine he practiced and knew I could work under him. Kate could work in Spokane and hospitalize at Sacred Heart. Not least, the offer solved our financial problem, which was that we had little money—certainly insufficient to start a practice on our own. Above all, it represented security. So why did I hesitate? Primarily because I knew I would be delivering the majority of the babies while the partners would be doing the surgery. Yet I had been in servitude for four years and their offer was an improvement. Why refuse a bird in the hand? I thanked my teacher, requesting time to decide.

Detail men, as they were then called, were salesmen for the drug companies. There were several based in Spokane and covering the adjacent territory. When I confided in one that we wanted to set up practice and needed him to recommend a location, he asked if I knew the TriCities. I replied that I had visited Richland and liked it, partly because of its climate, warm enough to swim while snow was falling in Spokane. He suggested that I look at Kennewick, one of the two smaller towns, which had no obstetrician or pediatrician and where the other doctors were congenial.

We had to reconnoiter Kennewick and soon, for I had only a month left. Kate and I arranged to meet there the following weekend. My guide recommended that I contact the leading GP, who was doing most of the obstetrics. I met Ralph at the hospital and found him to be charming from the first moment, taking us around the thirty-bed Kennewick facility. We dined with him and another GP, Brian, both fifteen years my senior. They noted we were not U.S. citizens and could not rectify this for two years; also, we lacked Washington medical licenses, though we were licensed in New York. (We were due to take the local exams in the fall.) We had practically no money.

Following this dismal discourse we stayed in a motel by the railroad tracks, feeling pessimistic about our chances. We reconvened at the hospital on Sunday morning with our two interrogators but now we questioned them, feeling we had little to lose.

Kate made rounds of the hospitalized children. She listened to their histories, examined them and discussed each case. She visited the nursery, inquiring about the care of prematures and making several cogent recommendations. Ralph showed me the delivery register, asking my views on several patients, and we examined the surgical log, discussing gyn cases. Over sixty babies were delivered monthly and the hospital census revealed occupancy rates near 100 percent. The medical staff comprised seven general practitioners, a surgeon, a radiologist and a pathologist. They had no internist, an alarming omission. The need for our disciplines was evident considering the delivery rate and number of pediatric admissions.

Our hosts conferred and Ralph told us that despite our statutory shortcomings, they would welcome us on the staff on July 1. It would be necessary that one of them countersign our hospital charts, and they would arrange with the pharmacies to honor our prescriptions. This probationary period would last until we had state licenses.

They made these assurances without scrutinizing our CVs or asking for references from our residencies, or even for the names of people to call. Ralph suggested we apply to the Sears Roebuck Foundation for a loan, because they assisted doctors in establishing themselves in rural areas.

Ralph became my last mentor, possessing an ability none of his predecessors displayed. He was a student of human behavior and the motivation that underlay it, sensing intuitively how you felt. This empathy was allied to liberal views, candor and a sense of humor. These virtues made him a fine doctor and a stimulating companion.

We accepted his generous offer on the spot and it was agreed that I would arrive on June 30, 1957. Kate would travel at night by bus from Seattle alternate weekends, see sick children in the hospital, and spend one day a month in the office during the last six months of the year, becoming full-time in January. We shook hands on this verbal agreement. No lawyers were needed and no documents were signed. This trust suffused our relationships with our Kennewick colleagues for the duration of our tenure.

I presented data to Sears documenting the need for a pediatrician and obstetrician in Kennewick. That was the easy part of our loan application. The budget was difficult. I asked for ten thousand dollars, as we had less than three hundred dollars between us. Obs and gyn were slow starters financially, because one had to wait until after the delivery for any payment, and surgery would be hard to find initially since patients liked to know a doctor before they trusted him to operate on them. Pediatrics is quicker to start but we faced six months' delay there.

Sears responded quickly, instructing me to meet an obstetrician representing them at a Kennewick motel the following Saturday. He was a shrewd man from Coos Bay, Oregon, where he practiced. He met privately with our two sponsors at the hospital, following which he questioned me on some obstetric cases. We studied the surgery log book and he asked me to comment. Returning to the motel, we discussed the budget, where it quickly became apparent that I did not know the cost of many items we should need, was ignorant of salaries and rents and other costs, and had little idea of current fees. As we parted, he promised a decision in three days.

The remarkable aspect of our meeting was what was omitted; namely, the contributions Kate would be making to the community as the only pediatrician. In common with many obstetricians of his era, he considered that pediatricians had little effect on what we had been discussing: the reduction of infant mortality and morbidity. The truth was then, and is now, forty years later, that advances in management of the newborn have had greater effect than those in prenatal care and delivery.

So he was Cyclops—but a helpful one-eyed giant. Sears' goal—to improve the health of a community by assisting doctors to locate in areas where they were needed—was a good and sensible one. Our loan application was approved, the budget reduced from ten to four thousand dollars, which we gratefully accepted.

Chapter 7

Indian Heaven

On learning of my desertion, my teacher was magnanimous, wishing me success in a risky venture and vowing to refer to me any of his patients who moved to the TriCities. I grandly reciprocated—an empty gesture since I had no patients.

I again packed our few possessions into the old VW and on June 30, 1957, rattled down to Kennewick, where it was hot—ninety degrees in the shade, of which there was little. I took a room in a shack motel by the tracks.

My first task was to hang a shingle. The doctors all practiced in purpose-built offices opposite the hospital, which they owned rather than rented, but I could not afford space there.

Apart from the hospital, the only area I knew was Angus Village. This section was at the crest of the hill above the Columbia River and adjacent to the country club and golf course, yet only two miles from the hospital. Newly developed at the intersection of two highways, the three blocks contained a motel, a bank, supermarket, drug store, and a variety of offices and shops. There was also a McDonald's, a novelty at that time, and a gas station and a café.

At the bank, I opened an account of $4,300, $4,000 of which belonged to Sears. On the strength of this I sought the manager's advice about renting an office and was told that Angus Village would be an ideal site for our purpose, as the surrounding area featured new homes and apartments, many occupied by young couples eminently at risk of becoming our patients. Indeed, the bank, a branch of the largest in the state, had surveyed the town and selected this location in preference to downtown. Grasping the fact that women were our prey, the manager ventured the opinion that they would find our office more convenient than the hospital, which was out of their way and not near the shopping district. He recommended that I meet with the developer who built the entire project, whose office was next door.

Frank was a Westerner, wearing a Stetson, check shirt, jeans and cowboy boots. We had several business dealings involving the office and our home, but never used a lawyer. An agreement and a handshake were always sufficient.

The first deal we made was modest, but critical to me. I put all my cards on the table, telling Frank our hopes, what little capital we had, and that Kate was delayed for six months. We walked across the courtyard, where he had two vacant adjoining offices that when combined would have enough space for our practice. They were on a corner, in front of the motel and next to the bank. Opposite was the pharmacy, and the hardware store was our neighbor. There were two entrances, one at the front and one at the back where we and the staff could park. We were the first occupants and the interior was unfinished, but there was plumbing, heating and air conditioning. Frank asked $200 a month rent, payments to start in January when Kate arrived, and I accepted with thanks.

Frank knew every subcontractor and recommended first a cabinet-maker, Wendell, whose skill proved invaluable. He also named a plumber, electrician, painter, floor man and sign painter. "You're in business, Doc, don't be shy," he urged. Put your names and trade in gold on the windows front and sides." I inquired where I should locate these craftsmen.

"That's easy, they assemble at 7:30 AM and again at 5:30 PM in the café"—pointing—"and when you show, they'll see breakfast, lunch and dinner."

Before we parted, he asked where I was staying, winced at the answer, and said, "I own a group of apartments, studios really, next to the golf club. They're full now, but I'll reserve one for you both for January 1. Meanwhile, I have an idea. Let's get in the car."

We drove two blocks to the club, where he showed me the apartments, small but convenient. "Then, there's a space we used as an office during construction. It's a store room now," he said, and showed me a basement room with a toilet and shower, a stove and sink, and a telephone. It was stifling hot inside, full of old wood and spiders. "It's yours for twenty-five a month, you pay the telephone. To keep cool, use a fan and leave the door open. It will be warm in winter under the earth. Got any furniture?"

"No."
"Go to Goodwill in Pasco."

In the dead of night, the telephone rang in my basement den and a doctor, whose name I did not recognize, asked me to come immediately to the Pasco Hospital. I had not visited the hospital nor had any contact with the doctors or the Catholic Sisters who governed it. The newspaper carried a paragraph noting my arrival so I concluded the doctor had seen this.

"When you first think of postpartum hysterectomy, it is already too late," is an adage and was the first thought I had on seeing the patient. She had delivered a large baby vaginally, her fifth, and continued to bleed after the placenta had separated despite the use of a drug that contracts uterine muscle. Her uterus was large and flabby, lacking tone, and I knew it was distended with blood. She appeared near death and, after performing a pelvic exam, during which I ascertained she did not have a uterine rupture, I asked the vital question, "What blood group is she?"

"O-Pos," the doctor answered. "I've sent for another bottle." One was dripping slowly in a small vein.

"Send someone to the lab, get another bottle and ask them to match all the other O-Pos they have, immediately. Put a larger line in her quickly before it is too late," I told the anesthetist. "Pump the bottle we have and then get ready for a general." Then I asked if the husband was there.

"Yes, he's outside. I know him well."

"Good, we'll tell him and then scrub. Prepare her quickly for hysterectomy," I instructed the obs supervisor. "Wrap her legs tightly before you put them down while someone else preps her."

Not unnaturally, the supervisor was reluctant to follow these instructions from a man she had never seen, who had invaded her delivery room, and who proposed to perform a hysterectomy on a woman in her reproductive years. Sensing her opposition, I said, "Let's try to save her while we have a chance instead of standing around watching her bleed to death."

We spoke to the husband, describing the crisis, my recommendation, the reason for it and risks involved. He agreed, and looked reassured that we were doing something.

When we returned from scrubbing, we met the Mother Superior. She had been summoned by the obs supervisor because of the gravity of the case and the drastic remedy proposed. When I explained quickly that no lesser course held hope and that death was the alternative, she accepted this readily and galvanized the OR staff with her commitment, authority and energy.

The patient survived. It was fortunate to meet the Mother Superior under these circumstances, and we became friends. (Postpartum hemorrhage such as this was responsible for the British abandoning home delivery. A patient like ours, following several normal pregnancies, appears low-risk, but the uterus, giving no warning, fails to contract after delivery. The resultant bleeding is continuous and life-threatening.)

Work progressed on our new office and we soon were able to open. What I had not anticipated was how well Kate's and my different disciplines integrated, resulting in an enjoyable and supportive atmosphere for patients and staff. Except for visits from the detail men, I was usually the sole male, invisible in my fastness at the back of the premises. Any men who accompanied patients to the office, overcome by the domesticity prevailing, retreated to the drug or hardware store.

Brian, one of my sponsors, visited the office. "I just want to tell you a few ground rules," he opened. "We have no evening hours and don't open on Sundays. We all see welfare patients, never turn them away, you deal with whatever problems they present, do not refer them on. All shots are three dollars, we don't want any two-dollar shots." I rarely gave shots but listened gravely. "We have a roster at the hospital, everyone except x-ray and path is on call for twenty-four hours, in rotation, for emergencies or walk-ins with no doctor; you see everyone that shows, you may keep the case or refer it. Staff meetings are at the hospital first Wednesday of every month at 7:00 AM All deaths and serious cases are presented." Then he relaxed. "Some advice—don't join anything. They'll ask you, just say no. You'll be too busy working to do anything else."

Kennewick is an Indian name that means "winter heaven." It becomes cold there and snows, but such conditions prevail only for a few days before a Chinook, a warm wind, arrives and melts the snow. Summer lasted until the World Series began. The annual rainfall was only seven inches, so we lived in a desert, with air that was dry and crisp. The visibility was remarkable. The Blue Mountains, fifty miles away, were clearly etched. Smog was unknown. It was perfect flying weather, cloudless all year. Irrigation overcame the aridity, making the gardens bloom and the golf course green.

The Columbia formed the northern border of town. A deep, cold, fast-flowing river, rising in Canada, it was joined by the Snake, out of Idaho, and the Yakima, a pretty local tributary. These three rivers conjoined just below the town, the surviving Columbia being over a mile wide. Pasco, the same size as Kennewick, was directly opposite and could be reached by two bridges, the old and the new across the Columbia. Twelve miles upstream lay Richland. This town was created during the war by General Electric and Dupont when the atomic bomb was built, and a group of nuclear reactors are sited on the Hanford Reservation covering a large acreage to the west.

The surrounding area, featuring tumbleweeds and jack rabbits, was divided into large ranches that grew wheat. There was farming in the valleys and blooming orchards. Yakima, eighty miles west, and Walla Walla, fifty east, were the nearest towns.

It quickly became apparent to me that one of the advantages of working in Kennewick, besides the weather and the natural beauty of the place, was Ralph, the local GP who had hired us. In a conservative and traditional community, Ralph's liberalism and elfin sense of humor were most refreshing.

The high school, library, and hospital were all situated close together and I stopped one noon in springtime to return some books on my way to work. Inside a car parked behind the building, two students were copulating. I reached the hospital in an indignant frame of mind, which Ralph immediately diagnosed.

"Why so worked up?" he asked.

I described what I had seen, adding, "It's disgraceful!"

"Oh I don't know," he replied, "it leaves their evenings free."

Once I got a speeding ticket following which I was called to assist Ralph in the OR, where I arrived in a bad temper.

"Why so distressed?" he asked.

"I got a speeding ticket."

"No, you didn't, you got a use ticket," he replied. "You buy a car, paying too much. You get tags, insurance, and an operator's license. All that stuff entitles you to drive the highways. When you do that, you periodically get a use ticket, for speeding, parking, running the light, or whatever. The more you drive, the more use tickets you get. It's a fair and logical system."

I often assisted Ralph in surgery. My compensation was supposed to be twenty percent of the surgical fee. On one occasion I helped him with an arduous case, a long procedure followed by a stormy convalescence during which Ralph often sought my help. Two weeks following her discharge Ralph greeted me morosely. "Do you remember the rancher's wife?"

"Yes, a struggle. Has she more complications?"

"No, she did well. Her husband came in with her yesterday, thanked me, wanted to pay. He's rich, thousands of acres, so I asked $500. He pulled out a bundle of hundreds and said, Ralph, you're a gambler, why don't we toss for it, double or quits, and…'"

"We lost."

"'Fraid so."

Once when Ralph and I were discussing changes in sexual mores, I detected a deviation from his liberal views, and tackled him: "Ralph, are you criticizing masturbation?"

He replied, "Certainly not, but you don't meet many interesting people that way."

Another time the local cinema proposed to show "adult movies." There was indignation and opposition, and Ralph was asked for his opinion. "It won't last. Coitus is a poor spectator sport," he responded.

My friend Brian's prediction that we would be too busy working to do much else was, not surprisingly, accurate. The only way we could leave town was to impose on Ralph for coverage and then repay him in kind. Before the children were born, we stole away for a weekend to visit Lake Chelan in a region known as "Little Switzerland." The lake is narrow, deep, and sixty miles long, enclosed by steep mountains set in a wilderness.

Following a long drive, we arrived in late afternoon at the southern end of the lake. It was spring and the motel had just opened for the season.

Kate said, "I'll drive into town, get some supplies, and case the place. You look hot and tired. I suggest a cooling dip in the lake followed by a nap."

Recognizing an order when I heard one, I put on my swim trunks and strolled across the motel lawn to the water's edge. The lake looked inviting, glinting in the sun just dipping behind the mountains. No one was swimming but there was a diving board and a raft floated about seventy-five yards from shore. Summoning my courage, I dived in, to discover the water was icy cold, almost paralyzing me, spurring me to swim as fast as possible before I froze. I am a slow swimmer, restricted to the breast stroke. When I reached the raft, I struggled to pull myself up and lay, grunting. Looking at the shore, which appeared far away, I saw the stout motel manager gesticulating, indicating a telephone as his voice carried across the still lake. "Doctor, hospital, emergency, woman dying," was the gist.

I was embarrassed to shout that I needed a boat to reach the shore. I flopped back into the deep, and fearing I was going to drown, swam literally for dear life back to the dock. Barely able to climb the ladder, I fell onto the lawn at the manager's feet.

"The doctor says a woman is dying, trying to have her baby," he said excitedly.

"Ralph's idea of a joke," I thought, staggering to our room still soaking wet. I lay on the carpet, blowing and gasping into the phone.

"I know what you've been doing," said the familiar voice.

"No, Ralph, you don't. Swimming. I've been swimming."

"Yes, of course, Dick, but so soon? I envy you, just slow your breathing down."

"I can explain."

"I'll bet, but let me explain that your patient needs a section."

"If you say so, she really needs one. Please go ahead. Thank you."

"O.K., just wanted to check. Glad to learn you are using your time wisely. Bye-bye."

Early in practice I had my first maternal death. Around midnight, I had a patient admitted in early labor. She was at low risk, having had an easy vaginal delivery less than two years earlier. I told her I would use a local anesthetic, a pudendal block, to provide pain relief during delivery, a technique I had used many times previously. I lay down in the doctors' room.

The nurse called me at about 4:30 AM The patient was cheerful, excited even. I held her hand and said, "Well done, we'll adjust the mirror so you can see what's happening and work with us." She was young and strong, with a big baby coming easily. I injected the anesthetic slowly and was just performing the episiotomy, when the head appeared. "Good," cried the nurse, "one last BIG push and you've done it." The mother raised her head in effort and grasped the nurse's hand. The baby shot into my lap. The mother gave a ghastly gurgle, her head fell back, flaccid. I cut and tied the cord, placing the baby on the receiving table. Directly I stood up and saw the mother's face, I feared she was dead. She was blue, not breathing, and, when I uncovered her, I could hear no heart beat and got no blood pressure.

"Shall I give a cardiac injection of adrenaline?" asked the nurse.

"Yes, let's try," I replied. But despite all our efforts, no pulse or blood pressure returned.

"She's had an amniotic fluid embolism," I said, "There's nothing more we can do. Is her husband here?"

"Yes, I sent him into the hall when we came into the delivery room. Shall I call him?"

"No, let me sew up the episiotomy and think. You care for the baby, she's getting cold. Stay in here, don't leave until I tell you."

I sutured the episiotomy, went to the phone in the sluice room and called Ralph. It was 5:00 AM He told me to stay where I was, speak to no one, he'd be there in five minutes.

I had seen amniotic fluid embolism result in sudden death before. The baby is surrounded by this fluid. Rarely, under high pressure, some fluid is pushed into the mother's bloodstream, where it travels to the lungs and causes instant death, just as a pulmonary embolus from a blood clot does.

Ralph arrived, agreed with the diagnosis, and we went together to meet the husband. I recounted what had happened and Ralph corroborated it. By noon, the husband appeared at the office. He was the beneficiary of a $20,000 life insurance policy on his wife, an unusual arrangement.

He asked me to complete the details of her death on the insurance form, which I did. My nurse told me he married the babysitter within a month.

Kate arrived in January 1958—just in time, for I had used all our money and borrowed all I could. I was certain that her personality and skills would attract many patients quickly, and gambling on that, everything was in the shop window, nothing in reserve. The office was staffed and equipped to handle large numbers of patients.

The first nurse to join us was Janet, who had been the only staff of a doctor who had recently retired. She had run his office singlehandedly—and, I imagined as I became aware of her talents, his practice as well. She was clinically experienced, knew everyone, and had a sly sense of humor.

Her laconic comment, "Gonorrhea on the hoof," introduced a self-styled cocktail waitress or a young lady of uncertain virtue and variegated background who was passing through town. Some patients were apprehensive over a pelvic examination and responded by wiggling up the table, delaying the proceedings until they were repositioned; one nervous lady moved repeatedly until finally her head was against the wall. Janet, losing patience, said, "If you go any further, we'll all be in the hardware store."

One of our patients had been married three times. Janet told me: "I don't know how she stands it. Training one man is hard enough. I couldn't start over."

I cared for a woman who lived seventy-five miles distant on a remote farmstead, whom I had delivered twice with no complications. She was now in her third pregnancy, which was a normal one. I entered the examining room, sat down, smiled at her, glanced at the chart, and raised my arm to touch the bell without having uttered a word. My patient grasped my wrist, saying, "No you don't, you listen to me and talk to me." That deserved rebuke taught me a lesson. I was hurrying so I had neglected the patient as a person, and saw her as just another case. After she left Janet asked, "What's wrong?" I told her.

"I should have warned you, she gets pregnant as an excuse to come to town and talk to someone. Can't blame her, marooned out there with a man who only knows how to…"

"I understand, thank you, but I must slow down, relax, and listen."

We had one family comprising a mother and her two daughters who confused me with their fecundity. I asked Janet, "Is it true that two of this family are always pregnant?"

"Absolutely, a house rule."

"I have just examined the younger daughter and I'm certain she is pregnant, and we just delivered her. If I'm correct, she conceived less than four weeks postpartum. That's a record. Have you taken a pregnancy test?"

"Yes, and we'll submit her feat as a record for the eleven western states."

"Janet, what can it be, it's not genetic. What do they share in common?"

"Same diet."

We needed another nurse and Janet suggested Bernie. They made an ideal pair. Janet was harder, cynical even; Bernie was soft, patient with new mothers and babies. They organized the staffing, set the schedules, and did the hiring (we had no firing) and, more important, the training. We employed only RNs, for we delegated to them all prenatal and well-baby care, contraception and post-op instruction, patient education and counselling, in addition to nursing procedures. They screened all telephone calls and called in prescriptions. The patients liked the system and would confide in the nurses when they might be reluctant to talk to us, especially to me. Patients frequently asked for Dr. Janet or Dr. Bernie, who were nurse practitioners before the term was coined.

We added a receptionist and a bookkeeper and a third RN, Mary. We also added part-time nurses when especially busy or for vacations. Our three first-team nurses all had their families complete, but the fecundity in our part-time nurses was remarkable. We offered free obstetric and pediatric care to our employees, but that was not the motivation—something about the atmosphere, all the maternity and babies must have been contagious, and I began to suspect that our office was recommended for any nurse who had difficulty conceiving.

We needed gowns for the patients and only green were offered locally, which the nurses rejected. They secured a supply of cotton gowns in a range of pastel colors for adults and children that were popular with the patients, who could request their favorite color. One patient who had been kept waiting on the examining table complained," It's boring to lie here looking at a white ceiling, can't you cheer it up?"

"Certainly, what would you suggest?"

"I'm an artist. I'll paint murals on the ceiling for you," she volunteered. So it was arranged. We provided the materials and gave her full rein without censorship, as we had faith in her artistic judgment. Her effort in the first room was extensive, colorful and complete. In the second, she was less ambitious and changed to an abstract theme, a lot of straight and squiggly colored lines. I suspected she had underestimated the labor involved and the strain on the neck and shoulder girdle consequent on painting the ceiling. But the result was that the rooms became more colorful and relaxing.

We soon found that new mothers had nowhere to put their babies while being examined by me post-delivery. The nurses who had to hold the babies enjoyed this, but were unable to perform their regular duties. Wendell, our cabinet maker, solved this, for his church had also faced a baby storage problem. He built four hutches with gates that could be closed, in which the babies were placed on a mattress. A space beneath provided room for their belongings. The infants were observed through the bars and were secure. They were adjacent to the play area in the waiting room, where the children enjoyed watching them. The pregnant patients could also see them, which improved morale. (Even I, an advocate of motherhood, admit that the later stages of pregnancy are tedious.) These hutches were a novelty, attracting the attention of our local newspaper. Finally, every space was put to use and the office proved adequate to handle at least forty children and twenty adults daily.

My promotion of motherhood was sometimes overly enthusiastic. The chief bank teller was important to us as she referred many patients. She had no children, attending only for annual checks, and on one visit she remarked, "I love seeing the babies in their little cages."

"Why don't you have one of your own then?"

"Oh, no, it wouldn't suit us. We've been so long without. A baby would disrupt our lives."

"Change them, you mean, in a wonderful way. Instead of being the eternal aunt you'll be a proud mother, fulfilled as a woman."

"Stop, Doctor, we are happy as we are."

"David would like it. Look at me, never thought I'd be a family man, now I pity men with no children to carry on their name."

Eventually, they had a fine baby but her life was ruined. Compulsiveness, which had served her well in the bank, made her a chronic worrier as a mother. She quit her job to stay home, where her child dominated her. As they quarreled over the child, her marriage appeared in danger. An intelligent woman, she lost her wits where the baby was concerned, constantly calling the office so that even Bernie grew impatient. When Kate said, "How dare you interfere with that woman's life? Women know if and when they want children. Why do you bully them?" I took the point and ended my advocacy of motherhood.

Working in the hospital emergency room was a lesson in prevention, for many of the injuries need never have occurred. One poignant case involved two young State Troopers who, on a Sunday, were practicing target shooting in a quarry outside town. They had a quick-draw contest and a revolver snagged on its holster, causing one man to shoot himself in the left femoral artery. His friend attempted to stop the blood without success, then struggled to carry him out of the quarry to their pickup. I was called to the hospital and found him DOA.

When in advanced pregnancy, Kate was summoned to the ER to find a man who had stabbed himself when attempting to kill a pig. The long narrow knife had penetrated deep into his belly but the entry wound was small. Seeing Kate, he said, "I don't want you, I want a real doctor."

"I am a real doctor and you're in real trouble," she answered. "You need an exploratory operation. I shall give orders which will prepare you for that and I will care for you until the surgeon arrives." Two years in Brooklyn inured one to insults from experts.

"You behave yourself," added the ER nurse. "You're lucky to have Dr. Kate, since she's accustomed to dealing with children. Now sign here." He did.

Kate used the telephone as an extension of her stethoscope, asking the mother to put the mouthpiece close to the baby's mouth. In that way she could listen to the character of the child's cry, and the rate and quality of the breathing, and recognize an emergency such as croup in a young baby. Later, because of the size of her practice and the consequent increase in pediatric admissions, we enlarged the hospital, adding a childrens' wing of six rooms.

We sat the state licensing examination, a written test with no clinical or oral component, and passed. By now, I had the knack, having acquired three licenses in three years. I reflected that I would be only seventy-eight years old when I was permitted to practice in all forty-eight states. (Ironically, sixteen years later I was appointed a member of one of the test committees of the National Board of Medical Examiners. My task was to construct questions that formed part of the examination taken by all graduating medical students, as a basis for securing a license in the state of their choice.) These annual exams had kept us studying, a forerunner of recertification. Family Practice had not then been recognized as a specialty, which it later became—and to its credit it was the first Board to introduce recertification. Years later, we were delighted to learn that Ralph had been the oldest doctor to become recertified by the Family Practice Board.

Ralph counseled us on practice, saying, "You can't please everyone. Some of the people will love you, a few will hate you." It is true that certain patients just don't like you. A gesture, a word, some unwitting slight, offends them, or they can't tolerate your manner. That is why we were taught to be ourselves—not to feign with patients, for you can't spend your life pretending.

I recall a patient in whom I diagnosed twins, quite early. I told her this made her a high-risk patient and offered some suggestions. She never returned following that first visit, going to another doctor. She delivered in the hospital, had complications, and died. When the case was discussed at staff meeting, the question was raised as to why I had not been asked to see her. The reply was that the doctor had asked if I could be called, but the patient had resolutely refused.

(I do not relate this to imply the outcome would have been different. The probability is that it would not, for many maternal deaths become irreversible before the danger is recognized.)

We organized prenatal classes for all women who were to deliver at Kennewick. These were free and were held in the high school one evening a week. The nurses conducted the prenatal care sessions and Kate taught newborn care. I did a session on labor and delivery and one on family planning, while the hospital organized a visit to the labor and delivery suite. A frequent question was, "How will I know when I'm in labor?" To this, my reply was, "Being in labor is like being in love. If you are in doubt, the answer is no. True labor, like true love, gets stronger."

Upon her arrival, Kate encountered opposition in the nursery from an old RN who ran it, one reason being that Kate measured the circumference of the newborn's skull and recorded it in centimeters. The nurse had not seen this done before and treated the procedure, and Kate, with scorn. Any orders Kate gave she opposed or ignored. Her attitude was, "Why should a twenty-six-year-old, pretending to be a doctor, tell me what to do, when I've had years of experience?"

This difficult situation was resolved by divine intervention. I was called in consultation for a fetus in severe distress and decided on an emergency section in the slim hope of saving its life. I felt anxious that I was imposing emergency surgery on a mother who had a fetus that might be dead or severely brain-damaged. My referring doctor was tense because he wished he had called me sooner, or perhaps not at all, for now we had precipitated a crisis. Kate joined us in the OR as I made the incision and then rapidly delivered the baby, handing it to her, feeling certain it was dead. An air of gloom pervades when a baby is born dead, particularly following a section. Kate's detractor the RN bore an expression that said, "I expected this, now you're really in a mess." I hoped Kate would take the dead baby out of sight to the sluice room while I closed the incisions and decided what we were to tell the parents. Instead, she placed the baby on the receiving table and sucked the mucous out of the nasopharynx. Then, with the assistance of a young RN whom she had been training, she extended the baby's head. Using the infant laryngoscope Dr. Apgar had given her in New York, she cleared the throat of mucous under direct vision. She then inserted a slim plastic tube into the trachea and sucked out more mucous, spitting it out of her mouth as she advanced the tube down. When the windpipe was clear, she blew gently down the tube in small puffs. Her assistant, with a stethoscope over the baby's heart, extended her index finger. As the two women faced each other above the baby's body, Kate continued gently blowing. It was now completely silent in the OR as we watched this drama while working. Suddenly, after what seemed like hours, the nurse moved her finger down—once, a pause, then again, slowly at first but repeatedly. The baby pinked up, Kate stopped puffing air into the lungs, watching the heart beat via the nurse's signals, waiting for spontaneous respiration to commence. Soon, the baby was breathing on its own and Kate extubated it. Finally, the baby cried. As the two women stood crouching over the baby, now clearly alive, the young RN said, "The doctor performed a miracle."

"No," the nursery RN corrected, "the Lord performed a miracle using the doctor's hands."

Be that as it may, victory and reconciliation were complete. Every newborn had to have its head measured and recorded, and Kate had a champion, for there is no fervor to match that of a convert.

A forty-year-old patient, who had been married twenty years, came to me with her first pregnancy, prompting Janet to comment that she was reaching the "last chance gas station." There is an expression, "precious baby," which fits this case. All babies are precious but here the stakes were higher. I was taught that age was no handicap provided that it was not accompanied by medical complications, which become more likely with age.

The woman was healthy, having no hypertension, diabetes, or other chronic illnesses. The only abnormality was that she had not conceived after many years of exposure but did so at forty. She proved an easy patient to manage and her pregnancy was uneventful. Labor started spontaneously at term and she was admitted about 2:00 AM. I went to the hospital and examined her. Everything appeared normal for early labor in a primipara (woman having her first baby). Contractions were regular and the head engaged. I saw her again at 7:00 AM; progress was slow but persistent both in cervical dilatation and, more important, descent of the head. I was uneasy but did not intervene by rupturing her membranes or giving her a drug to stimulate labor. I examined her periodically while I was in the hospital and slow progress continued. I saw no reason for a consultation, which in practice meant talking with Ralph, unless progress ceased. We could then decide whether to stimulate, rest, or section her. I left for the office about 2:00 PM, directing the nurses to check the fetal heart rate every 15 minutes and to call me if it should vary from normal. I would return at 4:30 PM and reassess her.

Just after 4:00 PM they called. Nurses give bad news reluctantly, in bits and pieces. "We are having a little trouble in hearing the fetal heart. At 3:45 PM it was O.K. but at 4:00 I couldn't hear it clearly. Donna thought she heard it but then said it might be a uterine souffle. We have turned her on her left side, given her oxygen and listened again. Her contractions are stronger, membranes still intact, B/P is—"

I interrupted, "Did you hear the fetal heart at your last try? Answer yes or no."

"Well, no, but—"

"Put in a large line, I'll be right there."

Arriving in the labor room I greeted my patient and listened carefully all over her belly, taking my time, but could hear no fetal heart nor sense any movement. I looked at her without speaking and she started to sob. I attempted to hold her hand but she withdrew and turned away. I examined her and ruptured the membranes. The fluid was clear, not green as it is in some cases of fetal distress. I listened again but heard no heartbeat.

Her husband was present and I told them that their baby had suddenly, inexplicably, died. I advised that the safest course was the hardest one for the mother to bear: that labor would continue. I anticipated she would deliver before midnight, at which time the cause of the accident might be revealed. The patient hardly listened, turned her face to the wall and would not speak to her husband or me. Following a dismal evening I conducted a joyless delivery about 11:00 PM.

The baby was term-sized and looked normal. The placenta was apparently normal, with no sign of insufficiency, which the pathologist confirmed. I then talked to the parents but it was a monologue, for the patient would not speak, look at me or let me touch her hand.

I did not resort to the lies frequently told patients; that the cord was overly long and thrice around the baby's neck so that when the baby delivered it strangled itself, or say that the baby was abnormal and would not have lived more than a day, or that "God gives and He takes away." I never thought these falsehoods eased grief or were therapeutic. But they were evasive and destroyed any trust between patient and doctor.

I told her first that it was nothing she had done or failed to do that contributed toward this tragedy. I said the only unusual feature was the twenty years of involuntary infertility followed by conception and I did not know what bearing this had if any. I admitted that had I performed a section in the morning when the fetal heart was audible the baby might have survived but that I found no indication to do so. Labor had progressed normally and she delivered in twenty-one hours, not abnormal for a primipara of her age. I explained that it was important to elucidate the cause, for she might again become pregnant, and I requested an autopsy, which was refused.

In the morning I learned that she had discharged herself. She never visited the office but we both attended the Episcopal Church so I saw her each Sunday. She always looked straight through me as if I did not exist.

This case affected me, as is evident from the details still etched in my mind. I was taught in England, "Never let the sun set twice on a laborer," and I had not broken that rule. I had followed Dr. Eastman's teaching but failed his test: "If a mother enters the hospital with a living fetus, she must leave it with a living baby." She had not, for I had failed to perform a cesarean section during the fourteen hours she was in my care with a living fetus. With hindsight, I should have sectioned her for failure to progress, but, section required having a consultant examine her, and writing an opinion. The only emergency sections approved were those with dramatic, usually late, indications, such as profuse bleeding or placental separation. The outcome for the babies so delivered was often poor, which was incorrectly ascribed to the procedure, whereas the damage was due to the delay preceding the section. At that time, a subtle indication such as failure to progress and fetal distress would not have warranted approval.

Electronic fetal monitoring (EFM), which provides a continuous recording of the fetal heart rate and uterine contractions, did not become available until many years later. Following its introduction, a debate ensued concerning the benefits, disadvantages and indications for its use. Studies showed that EFM increased the C/S rate and, because of the false positive diagnoses of fetal distress generated by the interpretation of the tracings, some operations were unnecessary. The majority involved in this controversy lacked long experience in the pre-EFM days. The more data you have, the probability increases you will reach a correct decision, whether you are a commander on the battlefield, a meteorologist, or an obstetrician. In my case, I believe EFM would have revealed an aberrant pattern.

This case was a watershed in the way I thought about obstetric complications. I now placed the fetus first and then considered the method of delivery, not the other way around. I must have been the only ob in the U.S. who spent twenty-four hours every day with the pediatrician to whom he had to submit every baby. I learned that Kate had no interest in the route of delivery, whether vaginal, spontaneous or forceps, abdominal or flown in by the stork. She wanted babies who were full term, not premature, and in good condition with high Apgars and no birth injuries. When these criteria were not met, I had to justify my obstetrical management.

In this situation, we became perinatologists before the term was used. In complications affecting our patients, it was simple for us to see the mother together before delivery. In toxemia, hypertension or diabetes, for example, where the uterine environment grew hostile as pregnancy advanced, we agreed on a delivery date that appeared to offer the fetus the best balance between prematurity and stillbirth. In cases of Rh incompatibility, where a conflict exists between the mother's blood and that of the fetus, the timing was difficult. Exchange transfusion after birth, which in Kennewick, only Kate was able to perform, was a recurring stress throughout our time in practice.

Obstetricians have been criticized for performing too many tests and cesarean sections, and displaying too little compassion. What is overlooked by our detractors is the result of our work. In the U.S., infant mortality (death in the first year of life), has fallen from 28 per thousand live births in 1953 to 8.0 in 1994, a 71 percent decrease in 41 years. Despite this reduction, the U.S. figure is higher than that for many comparable countries.

A paradox exists. The U.S. has the best survival record for babies of any weight because our nurses and doctors are partners in high-risk obstetric and neonatal units using advanced technology, yet we trail other countries in infant mortality. This is because the U.S. is handicapped by the frequent occurrence of low birth weight babies—that is, weighing 2,500gms (5-1/2 lbs) or less. This situation has persisted since 1953 at seven percent of babies born, despite great improvements in other health and social indices.

Some countries have low birth weight rates of four percent, which ensure their infant mortality rate is lower than ours in spite of our professional and technical excellence. These countries have smaller and more homogeneous populations than the U.S. and provide prenatal care and delivery with fewer access barriers.

In summary, we have too many babies born too soon, too small. We must keep these fetuses in the uterus longer. Despite many and various efforts, which initially showed promise, this hurdle has proved intractable to surmount. It is more than a medical problem, it requires changes in political and economic policies, and cultural and social attitudes.

It was snowing when Kate was ready to deliver following an apparently normal pregnancy. She took the train to Spokane while I remained at home. Two days later she reported that our son, James Ferguson Morton, named for my father, had been born. She said that on examination, a congenital defect had been discovered in his pelvis and she was discharging herself from Sacred Heart Hospital to take him to Seattle Children's Hospital. There he would be seen by a pediatric surgeon. Thus started a nightmare from which I expected to waken but it was reality. I did as requested, stayed home, ran the practice and took care of Nancy, our firstborn now fifteen months old.

Pediatric surgery was in its infancy and the surgeon was the only one in the Northwest, whom Kate had known when she was at the hospital three years earlier. The pathology involved the bowel, and after several operations were performed, Kate brought James home. She and Eleanor, our housekeeper, cared for him, and Kate attended the office for brief periods. When complications occurred, she took him back to Seattle for more surgery, then brought him home, and this sequence was repeated. This agony continued for four months until he died at home.

We had every advantage. We had knowledge, immediate access to expert care, special privileges, money, support from one another, and a healthy baby at home. How parents lacking these assets cope, I cannot imagine, for the ordeal was unrelenting. Alternating hope and despair, twenty-four-hour stress, fatigue, unending inquiries, curiosity and sympathy, waking up and facing the nightmare, railing against fate—what had we done to deserve such punishment, what sin was unforgiven, blaming one another, wishing he would die and then looking into his eyes and realizing he knew your voice or touch—these are some of the memories that remain after years of suppression. Kate was depressed, insomniac, losing weight, her abundant energy drained.

When it was over, Ralph told me I must take her on vacation. I protested, "We can't leave, what about the practice?"

"We'll look after that, Kate needs to get away now."

Ralph instructed me. "Fly to San Diego, get a car, drive to La Jolla and stay at this motel."

Kate agreed passively, unusual for her. It was late March, cold and windy in Kennewick. The motel was south of La Jolla right on the beach, with few visitors for it was out of season, but it was balmy. A sea mist in the morning dissolved by 10 o'clock, the remainder of the day being sunny. We walked on the beach and were able to discuss James's death and the deformities that caused it. Kate explained that their pattern did not conform to any syndrome of genetic or hereditary origin. Rather, they were consonant with an environmental insult to the embryo such as infection. She recalled a transitory illness with fever early in pregnancy which she ascribed to a virus contracted from a child she was treating. This would account for the gut deformities if the virus was circulating in her blood during the early development of the intestine. This etiology was cogent, for it meant that future pregnancies would not be at increased risk, compared to those of similar couples without such history as ours.

We relaxed, recuperated and enjoyed ourselves for the first time that year. La Jolla Cove is delightful, and once we dined at the Valencia Hotel, situated above a series of terraced gardens overlooking the ocean. Kate slowly recovered her health and spirits, in ten days wanting to go home. Owing to the generosity of our colleagues, particularly Ralph, we were able to resume our life and work.

In 1959 I fell in love for the second time. It happened as I was driving the old VW home from Walla Walla on a now-forgotten errand. I rounded a curve and there she stood—ravishing, provocative, flaunting herself, the sun glistening on her curves. She made no sign, for I was already besotted. With indecent haste I made a U-turn, parked and walked unsteadily toward her, wearing a stupid grin. The new white Porsche coupe was mine in minutes, her owner surrendered her virtue for a signature. Where was prudence? Thrown to the winds, impetuosity ruled. No test drive, no comparison shopping, no bargaining, no reflection. Our faithful friend was abandoned, all her economical miles of faultless service forgotten, her fate uncertain—left, crestfallen by the roadside, her master not sparing her a backward glance.

My new love responded to me immediately, accelerating smoothly through the gears, signalling me her wishes by the tachometer. We entered the first turn too fast but showing her pedigree she gripped the road, pushing my body like a small plane banking, the suspension compensating as we swept flawlessly out of the curve thanks to her innate virtues, certainly not my skill. When I first braked hard the feeling was uncanny, as if a giant hand had reached from the sky and corralled me to a halt.

Nearing home, I was assailed by trepidation, coupled with guilt. Kate, showing no surprise, asked, demonstrating her prescience, "Will it take the baby buggy?"

As we became acquainted I explored the Porsche's limits and my own. The terrain was ideal for fast motoring, being sparsely populated and flat, with long straights through the desert. The car was stable at 115 mph indicated, tracking true with no nose lift.

Porsche drivers acknowledged one another then but sometimes riffraff of the road such as Jaguars and MGs had the insolence to signal us. We ignored them.

Kate gave me a white motorcycle helmet and asked me to wear it on all trips out of town. The first use was inauspicious. I was returning from Spokane at night, knowing every feature of the route, anxious to reach the hospital and check that no patient of mine had been admitted in labor or as an emergency during my absence. The first hazard was a small town, Cheney, which had a reputation for ticketing any vehicle exceeding 30 mph. I crawled sedately through it as midnight struck and then, free of this and convinced mine was the only car on the road, I sped south, taking the Porsche up to its limit. Reaching another small settlement just north of home I slowed, dawdling through it, when a cruiser appeared in the mirror, red lights flashing. I stopped and got out.

The trooper spoke to me but I couldn't hear due to my new helmet. I struggled to undo the straps but they were tight and unfamiliar. My opponent was shouting and suddenly there was a loud bang and a hissing sound behind him. He drew his pistol, my helmet finally shot off and rolled on the ground, and I yelled, "Don't shoot, your radiator hose has burst and I'm Dr. Morton." We were standing between the vehicles and I was facing the patrol car, from which gouts of steam emerged. He sheathed his gun, opened the hood, and asked for my papers, which were all in order. "Why have you stopped me, officer?" I asked innocently, "I was driving slowly."

"You're crazy," he replied. "I picked you up in Cheney because I'd never seen a Porsche going so slowly and thought it was stolen and you hadn't figured out how to drive it, then I lost you and have been doing 120 to catch you, and now you're crawling again. I'm going to take you in. What did you say your name was?"

"Dr. Morton, of Kennewick. I'm called to the hospital there so I, er, hurried but I'm always careful in towns."

"Is your wife a doctor?"

"Yes, a pediatrician."

"She cares for our little girl and my wife likes her," he mused. "Let's forget it. Go home slowly."

"Thank you officer, but I hate to leave you here disabled."

"Just get the hell out! I'll manage, Doc."

I raced only once, during a trip to Seattle. Snoqualmie Pass across the Cascades culminates in a long flat stretch on top where youngsters in souped-up cars would wait for an opponent. As I passed, a Chevy, powered by a big V-8, challenged me. On the straight, I had to redline the Porsche to keep them in sight, but down the steep slope (two lanes westbound only) the road curved sinuously in a series of zigzag bends, dropping steeply. There were many bridges with stone abutments where the two lanes narrowed to one. This suited my car and once I gained the lead their power was of no avail. Superior road holding, steering, and braking prevailed. Reaching the plains, we motored sedately, the kids waving at me, one in the back playing bongo drums. I thought, they're fifteen and fancy free, I'm thirty-seven with children, a pregnant wife, seven employees and a large practice for which I am responsible. That trooper was right, I was crazy—but, no more, I quit.

After attending a meeting and staying overnight in Seattle, I reached home the following afternoon, checked the hospital and arrived at the crowded office for the afternoon appointments. Janet greeted me. "The chief state trooper wants to see you."

"Who?"

"Major McCormick, the big red-headed Irishman. He's head of the whole shebang there," pointing to the State Patrol Office at the highway intersection, two blocks from ours.

"To see me?"

"Yup. Two years in the slammer, shouldn't wonder," she answered with relish. "Don't worry, time will pass just like that," snapping finger and thumb like a pistol shot, "We'll manage without you. State pen is at Walla Walla, convenient, nice easy drive. I'll come and visit you. He's got his cap on, that's standard procedure when they are going to make an arrest."

"Janet, say I can't see him. Say I'm..."

"You must see him now. Remember that nervous Nellie that went into false labor last week, you had to get up at two?"

"Yes, yes, what's she got to do with it?"

"Well, he's taking up half a bench in the waiting room and staring at her, she's hyperventilating already. Get it over with or she'll deliver in the office."

"She's hyperventilating, what about me? Hold him off. I gotta make a call."

"No siree, one Major—rare—coming up."

I'm finished, I thought, they got my number. A hundred ten miles an hour in a forty-five-mile zone, reckless driving, endangering minors. Maybe there was an accident, leaving the scene, evading arrest and worse. Seattle has called and because of my prominence he's here to arrest me. How did they get me? Caught the kids, I expect, they want to cop a plea so they gave me to the cops. No, maybe it was that guy in the station wagon full of kids, with his wife nagging him. I cut him off before the bridge, scared him, he was shaking his fist and cursing me, understandably—he got my number and reported it. What shall I do? I'll tell him the car was stolen—no, that won't do, I didn't report it and it's out back. I'll tell him I was never in Seattle, didn't go over Snoqualmie, it was another white Porsche, mistaken identification. No, that won't wash, they'll check the meeting and the hotel. I'll call Hugh now [the hospital's and our attorney]—no, that will make the Major certain I'm guilty—what was the drill, name, rank and serial number—172443—I remembered that—I'm going nutty—I—"

Janet intoned, "Major McCormick to see you, Doctor."

He was wearing his cap. He filled the patients' chair, had to lift his holster in order to sit down. As he leaned towards me, gun belt creaking, I backed away but we were eyeball to eyeball.

"Doc, what's this?" he asked, pointing to a skin lesion on his right cheek.

"That," I answered weakly, "that, Major, is commonly known as a rodent ulcer but correctly termed a basal cell carcinoma, an early skin cancer. They occur on exposed sites, more frequently in persons with a fair complexion such as yours, and on those whose work subjects them to sunlight for long periods, as you have been during your lengthy and distinguished career. When did you first notice it?"

"About two or three months ago. My wife tried various ointments but they didn't help."

"No, they wouldn't, skin cancer does not respond to that kind of treatment. Please remove your cap so I may examine your scalp and hairline. Thank you, that's much better. I see no other lesions but you must keep a watch. I shall refer you to a plastic surgeon in Spokane, who will confirm my provisional diagnosis with a biopsy and will excise the tumor with a margin of healthy tissue around and beneath it. Then he'll repair the wound in a cosmetic manner. Post-operative surveillance is important, for other cancers may occur in the same area. You will have to restrict your sun exposure."

"That will be easy, I'm desk-bound now."

"Happens to all of us, Major. No excitement any more. I'll call Spokane, tell them you're a VIP and must be seen this week."

"Thanks, doctor, I'll be there, when shall I return to you?"

"That won't be necessary. I'll receive a report but they will do all the post-op care. You have an early cancer, it's accessible and you will enjoy a complete cure."

"Thank you again, Doctor, you put my mind at ease."

"I know just how you feel. My pleasure. Good day."

Janet asked, "When's his next appointment?"

"Never," I replied. "He won't be coming back."

"Pity," she commented, "Bernie fancies him. She gets bored now and then, seeing only women patients. He didn't charge you, what shall we charge him?"

"No charge, please tell him so. I like to help my fellow men."

"Of course, and it doesn't hurt to have a friend at the top in the State Patrol."

"Janet, you're a cynic. Such a thought never occurred to me. Now to work, let me see Nervous Nellie. I feel sympathetic towards her, why, I cannot imagine."

That evening I drove the Porsche for the last time. To my friend the VW dealer, who said, "Getting old, Doc, can't handle it?" I explained, "It's too small, I need plenty of space for a growing family."

"Space?" he answered, "Why, I've got just the thing for you, a family man. Brand new, just in, nothing but space." With that, I moved from the sublime to the ridiculous as I drove the green VW bus home.

Kate was delighted with both the departure of the Porsche and the arrival of the bus. As I left for the hospital she exhorted, "Don't speed in our new bus."

"Don't worry," I replied. "The limit is thirty, the distance 1-1/2 miles. The bus can't reach thirty in 1-1/2 miles. We are safe."

And so we were for sixteen years and 200,000 miles. We sat up front like Ma and Pa Kettle, looking over the cars beneath us. When Kate needed to minister to the children she didn't have to slide over the front seat as in a station wagon, but walked back to dispense justice and care. The bus was the vehicle remembered by the family with affection, the setting of many stories.

A local man bought the Porsche and did not have decency to take her out of town. Worse, he was a club member, parking in the lot. When I saw her, it was as if she were my ex-wife who had not been "as faithful as a bird dog or as kind as Santa Claus," yet was glamorous, alluring, exciting, and still roused desire.

Her fate at his hands distressed me. "It's willful neglect, she needs a wax job. He's put Michelins on, not the best choice. A luggage rack—that's the last straw." Thoughts like these troubled me. Within two years, the car left, but not the yearning.

Ethics are illuminated more sharply in surgery than in medicine, for the rewards are larger and the temptation greater. I was called around midnight to the Pasco Hospital to assist Guy, a surgeon. There was a hobo jungle in the switching yard, and a derelict had been admitted after being stabbed in a fight. His belly had been ripped open, his intestines were severed, and blood and feces were present in the wound. He was an alcoholic, a heavy smoker, and obese.

When repairing the bowel, Guy placed small interrupted sutures meticulously, reconstructing the anatomy precisely. Then, preparations were made to drain the abdomen from three sites.

It was past 4:00 AM before we began the closure and I had a difficult case at 8:00, which was worrying me. I needed to put my head down, if only for an hour. Closing is lengthy, so I had a brilliant idea. "Why don't we use heavy wire, let him close by secondary intention, that way we'll be through in less than thirty minutes. He's already been under more than three hours. He is a poor risk, his liver is shot, his lungs are lousy, if we push our luck he may not come out of it. We've repaired the damage, let's quit." What I was proposing involved closing the entire wound in one layer with three or four heavy wire sutures. The convalescence is protracted and painful, the healing uncertain, but it is quick.

The anesthetist woke up and looked cheerful. The nurse called, "Get the wire." But Guy replied, "That's one solution, Dick, but he'll do better with a layer-by-layer closure. First, we'll lavage to control infection, then place three stab drains and put a pump on one. Is he stable?" he asked the anesthetist.

"Yes," came the reluctant reply. So we worked for another two hours. The sun came up, coffee percolated, the news came on the radio, all hope of sleep was lost. Had we been operating on the President, we could not have bettered the procedure.

I wanted to say, "Guy, we're only getting this bum fit enough to resume drinking and fighting, he's no good to himself and a pain to everyone else," but I refrained, for I admired the standards by which he practiced, which I would never reach. Instead, I asked, "Guy, how do you get these interesting patients, this is our second this year?"

"My name is burnt in one of the trestles of the overpass," he replied.

Our hobo recovered and, no doubt, rode the rods south to winter in California.

We were appointed consultants by the Washington State Adoption Society in our area. This meant that they referred couples to us whom they had approved as adoptive parents and women who had contacted them signifying their wish to place their babies for adoption. The State governed the adoptive process and the regulations ensured an equitable arrangement for both parties. The two crucial safeguards were that no agreement could be entered between the mother and the adopter before the baby was delivered. This prevented financial inducement or coercion. The second was that the mother could not surrender her baby until after delivery and a hearing before a judge. A third stipulation was the screening of the adoptive couples by the agency. As a result of these measures, the adoptive system appeared to be as fair as could be devised.

Women who wished to give up their babies were sent to us by the agency, but a greater number came to us directly and we referred them to the agency, then cared for them. In either case they fell into two groups.

The majority were young, twelve to seventeen, single, in their first pregnancy, in school or had dropped out. The second group were older, separated or divorced, with teenaged children. They often came from out of state and had moved temporarily to our rural area, where they had a relative. All the mothers were conscientious, attending prenatal visits, though often registering late.

When the baby was delivered, a light general anesthetic was used and the infant was taken from the delivery room before the mother awoke. I talked to the mother after Kate had examined the newborn, telling her it was healthy, but did not reveal the sex, reasoning that in the future, when she saw a child of the same age, she would not be so readily reminded of hers. In practice, few mothers asked the sex but when they did I gave the reason stated. If the sex affected her decision, I told her she could ask at the hearing and it would be revealed.

After the mother was delivered I notified the hospital lawyer. Both of the two judges at the courthouse lived in town and one of them came to the hospital after hours, together with the lawyer, and a hearing was held in the mother's hospital room. The atmosphere was gentle and friendly. The judge first asked the mother to identify herself, then asked whether anyone had persuaded, bribed, or forced her to surrender her child. Satisfied on these counts, he inquired if she had changed her mind since her baby had delivered, explaining that her decision would be irrevocable. Then papers were signed and witnessed. I do not recall a mother altering her decision. Perhaps this was due to the safeguards and the explanations given by the agency and reinforced by us.

The mother was discharged as early as possible and urged to keep her postpartum appointment and subsequent contraceptive visit. The local youngsters, pushed by Mother I suspect, did so; the older women we rarely saw again.

Kate kept the babies longer than customary, to observe them for problems. When satisfied, she discharged them. The adoptive parents did not collect them, for confidentiality was preserved. The lawyer's wife, who had five children, came for the child and the transfer was made later. The birth certificate was issued in the names of the adoptive parents. No attempt was made to match the baby to the adoptive parents.

When you need a doctor, like a policeman, you can never find one. That has not been our problem. We suffer from a surfeit of doctors. During the latter part of a pregnancy, Kate accompanied me to an obstetricians meeting near Portland, Oregon. The attendance reached 300, filling the hotel, and naturally our Portland hosts were well represented.

We had left home at dawn on a Saturday and made a fast trip in the Porsche. Kate decided to take the day off from medicine and joined the ladies program, which visited the Rose Gardens, followed by an extensive tour of money-wasting emporia. She returned from the ordeal tired and frustrated, as her silhouette did not conform to haute couture.

I managed to stay awake during the scientific sessions and we attended a cocktail party hosted by a pharmaceutical company, followed by a banquet at which we shared a table with some friends from Portland. The evening concluded with dancing and it was midnight when we fell into bed, exhausted.

About 3:00 AM on Sunday morning, Kate woke me. "I'm in labor, feel these contractions." Placing my hand on her uterus, I felt them to be moderate and regular.

"Fetch an obs," she demanded.

"I am an obs," I retorted, "you need to rest and I will observe the contractions."

"Until I deliver I presume. I want another opinion. The hotel is full of obs. Wake one up."

"I can't do that. What am I going to say? '"My wife is in pre-term labor because she ran around all day, shopping, and spent the evening drinking and dancing while I encouraged her. Now I don't know what to do, please help me?'"

"Call the university hospital then."

"No, the only person awake there will be an intern and they're dangerous."

"Call a private hospital then and get me admitted."

"No, all the competent obs are here."

"That's what I said. Wake one up."

"Shhh—not so loud, please, darling, you'll wake someone."

We had completed a round of circular reasoning and, in the diffident English manner of discussing quietly rather than making a nuisance or, worse, a spectacle of ourselves, had done nothing. I felt Kate's uterus again. "The contractions are no stronger, dear. I don't believe you are in labor."

"How do you know, you've never had a baby or a labor pain for that matter. True labor, true love, false labor, false love—what rubbish."

"Agreed, but it sells well."

"You don't know, can never know, what it's like. If I say I'm in labor I am until you prove otherwise."

"That's right, and time has proved otherwise so far."

Despite my arguments during this pillow talk, she had unerringly hit upon a crucial weakness, a failing I could not redeem. I fell silent, a signal of defeat in our discussions, then I surrendered completely, falling asleep. I was awakened a second time as Kate whispered, "Hey, don't feel badly, all's well and it's morning. About half an hour after you fell asleep they stopped. You were right."

Following a harrowing night we presented a united front. "How did you rest?" inquired Kate's friend at breakfast.

"Like a top, thanks," Kate answered, "and you?"

We decided, with no discussion, to leave early, and drove slowly home.

Abortion was illegal but a steady demand for it existed. I was asked to abort patients for the first time when I reached Kennewick. I explained that I could not, for it would result in imprisonment and losing my license. Patients disbelieved me so I said, "Kate and I are in the life business, Arthur Mondheim is in the death business." (He was our mortician, a competent, honest and sensitive friend. He sent us the largest bouquets for Christmas, and at the bottom of each basket, hidden among the flowers, was a bottle of brandy, for medicinal purposes.)

I felt angered by the need for abortion because it represented a failure in prevention, which was a cornerstone of our practice, contraceptive instruction being offered to all our patients. But, perversely, I sympathized with those so desperate to abort they were prepared to imperil their reproductive future and risk their lives in a clandestine, criminal activity. Several women told me they were going to Seattle to have an abortion. I suggested they contact me immediately after they returned home. Then I could examine them and limit the damage by a D&C, removing the placental tissue that usually remained, infected, in the uterus. Once the embryo had been destroyed and expelled and the pregnancy test negative, it was not illegal to treat an incomplete abortion; indeed, it was indicated.

Some patients related their adventures. One, I remember, involved visiting a department store and going to a specific stall in the toilet adjacent to the café. A message would be hidden there to be retrieved by the patient, specifying a corner in downtown Seattle where she should wait, wearing or carrying something distinctive, also specified. A woman would then meet her and lead her to the abortionist's office. This was located in a nondescript room where, after she had paid $300 cash, an abortion would be performed. The woman would then be left to find her way home, bleeding and cramping. The subsequent legalization of abortion in the U.S. reduced maternal morbidity and mortality.

I once cared for an athlete, a nurse who worked for us part-time, whose first pregnancy followed shortly. I diagnosed twins. She was a tall, muscular woman who told me she had swum for the U.S. during the last Olympics. I suspected then that I was merely along for the ride, because to reach such a pinnacle you need an iron will and belief in yourself. I knew she could manage her own body and any constraints I suggested would be ignored and counterproductive. Twins are a complication and I usually limit activity during pregnancy but I decided to observe and not interfere.

She and her husband, a physicist, were both Californians. Their family included King, a German shepherd.

Early in the year, when she was in mid-pregnancy, I remarked, "You look terrific—where did you get that tan, Hawaii?"

She laughed. "No, on Mt. Rainier. We just climbed it."

"Isn't it still deep in snow and dangerous."

"Sure, that's the point, but we know a couple of Rangers. They'd OK'd the climb."

"Do you sleep out?"

"Yes, as near the peak as possible so you can reach it at sunrise."

"How do you keep warm?"

"In the sleeping bag, and King lies by me. His coat is thick."

"Did the twins bother you?"

"Only because I had frequency and had to keep getting up and King kept me company. He had to urinate after me, in the same spot. It's a masculine canine prerogative, I guess. So it took time and I got chilled."

She and her husband belonged to the country club. One Saturday afternoon at the beginning of summer, when the pool had just been filled with cold water, I was sunning myself at poolside. I was the only male. The other guests were a bevy of society matrons—wearing sports clothes, seeking a tan, and gossiping.

My patient, in late pregnancy, appeared, wearing a swimsuit and carrying all before her in the shape of twelve pounds of fetuses and accompanying maternal support systems. The gossip ceased upon her entry, replaced by a rustle of disapproval and looks of condemnation. Ladies in her condition did not wear swimsuits, it was not maidenly. If they did so presume, they sat with their family in a discreet spot away from the limelight. She was an affront, furthered by her greeting me with "Hi, doc," and a smile. Watched covertly by her seniors, who feigned lack of interest, with no preliminaries she entered the pool with a flat racing dive, splashing cold water near the spectators. She swam the crawl with the precision of a machine. Powerful pulls of her arms were synchronized with her legs in a rhythmic beat as her body cleaved the water. Her breathing was methodical and controlled—inhale, exhale—her head turning, then submerged. No splashing or thrashing, no wasted energy, the minimum resistance to the water resulted. She executed the flip turn so quickly that I could not distinguish the different components. The first minutes were warm-up, then the rate increased to cruise and I lost count of laps. As time passed, the spectacle became hypnotic, boring; one forgot that a woman's effort produced it. Then, for several laps, the speed increased, the turns were urgent. I sensed she was striving for the old marks that would elude her forever. She relaxed and performed a medley, butterfly, back stroke and breast stroke, culminating with that burnished crawl. Disdaining the ladder, she abruptly pulled herself up with one easy lift, shed her cap, shook her hair down and gave me a big wink and farewell wave. I left surreptitiously, not wishing to be interrogated by the ladies' court, who were now pronouncing a guilty verdict. She was a pioneer in the athletic emancipation of women, which has demonstrated that gender is no barrier to record achievement in sport, and she vindicated my faith in her by delivering with no problem.

 In the course of my career I have treated more than a few eccentric patients, answered my share of off-the-wall questions, and found myself in less than dignified situations.

 At our clinic in Kennewick, new patients disrobed completely and were then attired in our pastel examining gowns. I would check them from their hair down to their feet. Some women applied perfume liberally so I got dizzy from the smell, but one patient presented a different hazard. I examined her heart and lungs, listening with the stethoscope. Then I palpated her breasts. While thus occupied, I was seized with a fit of sneezing. I retreated, recovered, and resumed the matter at hand, but with the same result—explosive sneezing followed by nose blowing, disturbing to both parties. I apologized, yet was puzzled, for I am rarely allergic. I doggedly approached her for the third time, whereupon she laughed and said, "It has the same effect on Roger."

"What does and who is Roger?" I asked, curtly.

"My powder makes my husband sneeze and I occasionally use it if I want to, er, deter him."

Our surgical patients were wheeled into the OR, sedated but awake, and anesthesia was induced there. One patient was about to undergo a hysterectomy when she intoned the Twenty-third Psalm: "The Lord is my Shepherd..."

The nurses ceased counting the sponges and arranging the instruments, and all stood devoutly still, with bowed heads. I was appalled, imagining the reaction in the hospital. ("Dick's patients are praying before he cuts them. You can't blame them.") Word would be around by lunchtime. I signalled the anesthetist, "Down, put her down!"

Thereafter, I asked my patients if they desired a visit from their minister prior to surgery and if they did, caused arrangements to be made.

When I saw a new gynecologic patient, Janet would accompany her to my office and introduce us. Sometimes, she made a comment to me alone beforehand. One day, she privately announced, "Mrs. Vanderbilt," in a society accent.

This dowager, expensively gowned, swept in, dripping condescension. "Oh Doctor, what a funny little office, hidden back here. I usually attend Dr. Big in Seattle, do you know him? No, well you're new here, from Brooklyn I understand. Now I have this annoying spotting, one might even say bleeding. You can see if it's anything important and then refer me to Seattle."

Another time, Janet introduced a new patient in Teutonic tones, "Achtung! Frau Berta from der Fatherland ist."

"O.K., please send her in."

"Jawohl, mein Herr—Sieg Heil!" A large lady in her fifties entered, with a forbidding expression, and sat down with a groan. Her guttural accent made interrogation difficult. She had many complaints, ranging from head to foot but centered amidships with a tendency to aft. Studying them I found no pattern except a lack of mobility. Her knees would not bend, her hips were fixed, to move in bed such agony was. Her female organs so tender were.

Pelvic examination was a struggle for all concerned, with grunting and sighing from the patient, exasperation from Janet. I took a Pap smear, and palpated the uterus and ovaries, which were normal. Having no diagnosis, I explained that I had taken a test that would provide valuable information. Suggesting she minimize movements that exacerbated her pain, I asked her to return in a week.

A week later, I found Janet perusing the lab reports before placing them in the patients.' charts, as usual.

"Anything interesting?" I inquired. Silently, Janet passed me a Pap smear report, folded so the name was obscured. It read, "Non-diagnostic specimen. The cervical cells are obscured by liberal deposits of spermatozoa. Suggest repeat test following forty-eight hours of continence." This implied that intercourse had occurred within several hours prior to obtaining the specimen, not rare as we had a young population.

"So what?" I commented.

Janet uncovered the name, Frau Berta.

"O.K., but I have to tell her something—what's the diagnosis?"

"'Scarcely at Death's Door,'" Janet responded dryly.

Another time, we had a premarital patient who was anxious and jittery. Janet taught her the diaphragm routine, which she practiced as a dry run before using it in action. But in the event, the patient later reported to us, all did not go smoothly. In the motel on her wedding night matters came to a head faster than our student had anticipated. She asked her ardent groom to wait a minute and hurried into the bathroom. Smearing the diaphragm liberally with cream as instructed, she put one leg on the toilet seat, reached the critical point of insertion, and was squeezing the slippery object when her beloved shouted, "Hurry up, for God's sake!" whereupon it shot into the toilet bowl. Unnerved, she was bending down trying to fish it out, when her husband pulled the door open and demanded, "Why have you got your head down the toilet?"

The emancipation of women, which has been the greatest sociological advance in my lifetime and the one that has given me pleasure to participate in and observe, is based on two factors. One is women's acceptance into education at all levels, in all disciplines. The second is the control of conception by hormonal means. Oral contraceptives removed, at one stroke, the biological yoke under which women had suffered for centuries. The new agent was revolutionary, for a chemical ruse deceived the pituitary gland into believing that conception had occurred, so that it suspended ovulation. Manipulation of the menstrual cycle by altering the normal ebb and flow of the hormones estrogen and progesterone was achieved by exogenous control, and no new elements were introduced into the system. The effect was temporary and reversible at will. OCs made barrier methods obsolete, both by their greater effectiveness in preventing pregnancy and by their independence from coitus in time and route of administration. (Despite the benefits they have conferred on women, OCs have not been universally accepted or acclaimed.)

I was fortunate to be asked by Syntex, a drug company, to participate in the early clinical trials of the OCs. We were provided with a protocol and the capsules. Eligible patients were enrolled and followed. I enjoyed the numerical aspect and recordkeeping and teaching involved; also, the study made a change from practice, which still occupied ninety percent of my time.

It proved difficult to convince some patients of the effectiveness of the pill because of its revolutionary nature. A patient whom I had delivered twice in quick succession was skeptical.

"You mean that if I swallow this every morning I won't get pregnant, won't need any other protection?"

"Yes."

"Fred can't get me pregnant any more?"

"Don't worry about Fred, the whole Marine Corps couldn't get you pregnant," I assured her.

"Doc, you've got to be kidding!"

This attitude was not uncommon. Some patients had difficulty with the regime, simple as it was, so we gave group instruction as many had similar questions.

"How do I remember to take the pill every morning?"

I asked "Do you do the identical thing every day on getting up?"

One woman appeared offended. "Naturally I do."

"Describe it, please."

"I open the kitchen curtains, of course." (The unspoken words were, "Doesn't everyone?")

"Then put the bottle on the shelf behind the curtains."

Frequent questions were: "What should I do if a) I forget to take the pill, b) I can't remember if I took it, c) I don't know if it's a pill day or not?"

One answer fits all: Take a pill.

Syntex inquired if I would be interested in joining their clinical research staff, based in San Francisco, to oversee trials at university hospitals. They asked me to visit. Kate advised me to talk to them, ascertain if they liked me and vice versa. As I was going to San Francisco I called a friend, a resident at Hopkins whom I respected, now on the faculty at UCSF medical school, and told him of the offer. His reply was concise— "Peddling drugs, prostitution of your medical degree." I canceled the appointment.

One surgical case, on which I never operated, gave me more concern than most of those on whom I did perform surgery. Jack was a G.P. who, excepting Ralph, was my best referral. He was a thinking doctor, a medical rather than a surgical type, who finally left to become a psychiatrist. He called me one evening.

"Dick, I've just admitted a young woman about whom I meant to call you earlier. She's only fourteen weeks but the uterus is already above the umbilicus. It has been growing rapidly since the start and I thought she had twins. She has been coughing, seems short of breath, is pale, with a fast pulse. She is not bleeding."

"Can you hear a fetal heart?"

"No, and that surprised me, considering the uterine size."

"What is the hematocrit?"

"It's low, about twenty-three I think."

"Ask the lab for three units of packed cells. Order an x-ray of her belly. Make sure they get all the uterus. Then get a chest film."

"Chest? Why?"

"Please, Jack, just do it, I'll explain later. Any relatives there?"

"Just her husband, he's a youngster. Her parents are my patients."

"Good. Call them in, please. Don't talk to them until we've met. Let's see, it is 7:00 PM, I'll meet you there at 9:00, we will have the films then and more from the lab. Goodbye."

There is a rare cancer named choriocarcinoma which is peculiar to pregnant women, for it is composed of chorionic cells derived from fetal tissue. The tumor is fast-growing, as it is composed of rapidly dividing cells. The uterus enlarges quickly, so it exceeds the growth rate in normal pregnancy and twins are suspected. As the embryo usually dies early, no fetal heart is audible. Tumor cells invade the uterine wall, but, worse, they spread throughout the body by the bloodstream, for the pregnant uterus has an abundant blood supply. Cells from the cancer spread to the lungs early, which compromises respiration, and fluid forms in the lungs from heart failure. The tumor is parasitic and the patient becomes anemic, adding to her cardiac problems. When lung deposits are widespread, death occurs from heart or lung failure. There was no effective medical treatment at this time by radiotherapy, or chemotherapy. These facts were in my mind as I listened to Jack.

When I saw the patient I was dismayed. She was propped up, both by the bedrest and pillows. She coughed intermittently, looking frightened and tired. She was pale, with a rapid pulse, no fever. The uterus was large, soft, and I could hear a uterine souffle as the blood pulsed, but no fetal heart. The chest film showed widespread tumor in fluffy snowflakes throughout both lungs.

I told Jack the diagnosis and pathology, adding, "There have been several papers recently demonstrating that if you remove the primary cancer from the uterus and do a pelvic clean-out, often the lung metastases regress and disappear, and the patient lives. Once the tumor is gone and no further cancer cells invade the lungs, the phagocytes (scavenger cells) deal with those remaining.

"If we do nothing she will die shortly. If we remove the tumor and uterus she may live, it's worth trying. Let's give her three units of packed cells slowly tonight and operate at 7:30 AM tomorrow."

Jack looked doubtful.

"Come on, we'll explain it to the relatives."

He introduced me to the husband and parents and I explained the predicament, showed them the films and recommended blood transfusion through the night, followed by surgery in the morning rather than waiting for death. The mother said, "We wish to talk to our doctor first before making a decision."

"That is wise," I responded, and left them.

Jack returned, looking gloomier than ever. "They don't like it, Dick, and I don't like it."

"We are unanimous then, for the patient doesn't like it and I don't either. But if we can get the tumor and uterus out, and I think we can, and if we can keep her alive through the procedure and subsequently, there's a chance—otherwise there is none."

"I understand that. So do they and they've agreed. I'll get the permissions."

"Thank you. I'll write the orders and tell Chuck (the internist)—we'll need him during and after surgery. I'll reshuffle the list and get some more blood lined up for tomorrow. We have a plan, let's stick to it. Get some sleep, I'll see you at 7:15 AM. Thanks for the case, Jack, interesting and a challenge."

"Save me from surgeons. Good night, Dick."

I was concerned over her fluid balance. I did not want to drown her by pushing too much blood pre-op, as her heart was already overloaded. But the procedure would be bloody and I did not want to lose her on the table from blood loss. It was a fine line.

I saw the patient again and conferred with the charge nurse on graveyard, who had good judgment born of long experience. "I'm glad you're on. Keep the packed cells running. She should go through the night OK. Got any suggestions?"

"No, I don't like it though."

"Join the club, the patient doesn't like it, nor do the relatives. Jack doesn't and I certainly don't. Listen, I'm tired out and strung up as well, it's nearly midnight. Please don't call me. Use your own judgment, you've been at it longer than I have. I need some sleep and once I'm woken I'll stay awake worrying."

"Understood. Good night, Doc."

At 4:00 AM the phone rang. "This is the ward," she said.

"Oh, I asked you not to call. What can't wait until surgery?"

"I think you need to know this before making the incision."

"The damage is done. I'm awake, tell me."

"She's dead, I'm certain."

Pause. "Where are the relatives?"

"Mother sent the old man home. She and the husband are asleep. I put them in an empty room."

"Don't wake them. Call Jack. I'll be down before he is. We'll see them together. Sorry I was rude, forgive me, please."

"Understood."

As I drove slowly through the darkness I thought, "You're lucky. If it had happened during or just after surgery, you would be in trouble. Now you are a prophet."

We gave our patients a book on prenatal care, labor, and delivery, followed by a book on child care. These books were popular and made our job easier, and we added one entitled *Ideal Marriage* for those who came for premarital counseling, which included family planning. This book was expensive so it was only to be loaned. All the books were inscribed with our names in gilt lettering.

I am, I discovered, a poor judge of character. A young woman visited the office, requesting a diaphragm fitting, which Janet did. When they returned to my office from the examining room I congratulated them on the speed and efficiency with which they had accomplished the task. Janet wore her inscrutable look. This patient must be intelligent, I reasoned, as well as demure and attractive, an ideal candidate to be the first recipient of *Ideal Marriage*. She accepted the book gracefully, promising to return it after she had grasped the contents. When I told Janet of my action she responded with a quizzical look and bit back comment, with some difficulty I fancied.

About two weeks later I received a call from the Chief of Police in Pasco. "Hi, Doc, have you lost anything personal in Pasco lately?"

"No, Chief, not that I can recall."

"Spent a night over here lately?"

"No, I live right on our end of the bridge. You know that."

"Spent an hour or two over here—on pleasure?"

"No, Chief, what's all the mystery?"

"Well, we just raided a cat house."

"A brothel!"

"I guess you can call it that but it's a well-run organization—caters mainly to the trucking industry."

"The what industry, Chief?"

"TRUCKING!"

"Oh, sorry, I misheard."

"It's one of a chain, based in California. They got places in Bakersfield, Fresno, one in Oregon and we, being a transport center and all, have one here." His voice rang with civic pride.

"They rotate the girls, see, gives them a change of, er, scene. But there's a conservative element in town to whom I have to cater, you understand. So, from time to time, close the operation down, make a fuss, the *Herald* reports it—good publicity for us."

"Yes, Chief, but what has this to do with me?"

"Well, Doc," we found a book with your and the Mrs. Doc's names on it, all in gold—*Ideal Marriage*—diagrams and all, an instruction manual belonging to a Miss French. Have you been instructing her, Doc?"

"No, no, she is a patient."

"Of course she is, Doc, of course. But if you want to see your girl—"

"Patient."

"Sorry, your patient, you'll have to be patient for a week. All the girls get seven days, see. Gives them a rest, no hassles, regular meals"—the Chief enumerated the virtues of incarceration—"and the management knows where their assets are at. But don't worry, Doc, by Labor Day the business will be running again, shouldn't wonder. Now me and the boys don't need this book down at the station house. One of my officers will drop it off to you."

"Thank you, Chief."

"All part of the service, Doc—see you in church."

Without any discussion, it was decided that I would delegate loaning *Ideal Marriage* to Janet. She returned the book to our shelves but not before sterilizing it twice.

Dancing once resulted in my being paid in song. A new band at the Club offered a wider repertoire than its predecessor. In addition to music for ballroom dancing, our specialty, they played Latin rhythms, country and western, and my favorite, Dixieland jazz.

The wife of the leader was the vocalist. She became my patient, suffering from chronic pelvic infection. I recommended surgery. She made a good recovery and her health improved.

Musicians lead a nomadic, precarious existence. Their employment offers no fringe benefits and they drift from gig to gig, sustained by applause and hope. She had no health insurance, no home and little money, but made a short-lived attempt to pay me. I did not press her. I had not cared for a singer before and seized the opportunity to discuss her art, the music and songs she liked, and to air my own preferences. (I cannot sing, play, read, or identify a note, but I enjoy music.)

I now realized I had my own chanteuse. For my conceit, I was paid in musical coinage, not bankable, and was pleased with the contract. For at the Club, the band played and she sang my favorites as we danced.

We cared for a thirty-five-year-old woman who had four children, the youngest of whom was mentally retarded. The mother, a large strong woman, presented in the seventeenth week of her fifth pregnancy, when I diagnosed twins. She developed false labor in the twenty-ninth week, and I asked her to stay in bed for the rest of her pregnancy. She was reluctant to do this, for she lived on a farm, where, in addition to caring for her children, she helped her husband. Kate talked with her and the unspoken word between them was that, with one handicapped child, every effort should be made to avoid a complication in this pregnancy. Despite our advice, the patient left undecided.

I was uncertain if rest would help, but feared that hard work would add to the risk of prematurity, a common complication in twins. So, the following day, uninvited and unexpected, I drove to the farm. I found our patient in the barn, using a machine to milk the cows. Her husband was maneuvering the beasts and toting bales of feed.

Overdressed in my dark suit, my gleaming black shoes covered in straw, I felt an intruder and an idiot but stuck to my guns. I explained to her husband that the next eleven weeks, and particularly the next seven, were critical for the twins to attain maturity. Every day, every week, that pregnancy could be prolonged was of value.

I asked if she would adopt bed rest as recommended by Kate and me. She said that they had not had time to discuss it, but it was plain that she had not raised the subject. Her husband promptly became my ally and they made arrangements for a relative to live in. I promised to make house calls but not on a regular basis, which my schedule did not permit; that ruse prevented the patient from hopping into bed just prior to my arrival.

I visited weekly and became a friend of the farmer as well as his wife. I learned the details of cow husbandry and a variety of agricultural matters. Labor developed at week thirty-seven, causing her to be admitted in the afternoon. Kate customarily attended twin deliveries but her office was packed, so I assured her that the twins were not preterm, that I would deliver them alone and that I would call her immediately.

Delivery was uneventful. The first baby, twin A, weighed 7 pounds, 1 oz. and the second, 4 pounds, 13 ozs. With Apgar scores of 8 and 7, they appeared fine to me. When Kate heard the weights she was excited, asking, "Is A purple and fat, and B pale and thin?"

"I don't know, what's that got to do with it?"

"Go back and look, you idiot."

"You're right, A is red and fat, B is pale and thin."

"Is the camera in your car?"

"Yes, I think so—why?"

"Go fetch it, we have a case of twin transfusion syndrome."

"What syndrome?"

"I'll be right there and explain."

This syndrome occurs due to a vascular anomaly of the twin placenta. One umbilical cord is larger than the other. Consequently, the fetus served by it (twin A here) is literally full of blood and larger than twin B, who is deprived of blood, being anemic and small.

Kate was concerned about twin A, which was stuffed with blood and had a hematocrit of 70 percent, whereas 40 percent is normal. The infant showed signs of heart failure and she performed an exchange transfusion, withdrawing 170 ccs of blood and replacing it with 140 ccs of fluid. Following this, the baby was pink and active. His hematocrit fell to 55 percent and he went home on the fourth day. His thin brother had a hematocrit of 40 percent and was an active, normal infant. At seven weeks, he developed severe diarrhea, and was readmitted with a hematocrit of 22 percent. Treated with intramuscular iron, he responded well. Both boys developed normally.

Kate wrote this case up in an article in 1964. Hers was the second case described in the literature, but the first where both twins survived. This was due to her having read and recalled the first article, recognized that baby A was in jeopardy, and treated him promptly and correctly. Twin births such as this must have occurred for centuries, but doctors had not recognized the condition. But for Kate, I would have paid no heed. She wrote in the article, "The striking clinical features of this syndrome enable it to be recognized at birth. One infant, the larger of the two, is ruddy and engorged with blood, with a thick cord. The deprived twin is smaller, scrawny and pale, with a thin cord. The condition should be borne in mind at all twin deliveries."

Twin transfusion syndrome and fetal alcohol syndrome are examples of conditions that were first diagnosed by observation. Fetal alcohol syndrome was first recognized in 1970 in Seattle by a woman pediatric resident. She observed, over a short period, four newborns with stunted growth and abnormal faces. These babies looked like each other but unlike normal babies. She noted that their mothers all shared a long history of alcoholism. From this description, the syndrome was defined and the causality established. Fetal alcohol syndrome must have existed since women first drank alcohol, yet it also had been overlooked.

This was an era when patients gave gifts. When a young girl died of leukemia after a long struggle, Kate, who was close to the patient and her mother, a farmer's wife, grieved. A month later, a man called at the home, asking for Kate. I explained she was at the hospital. "Then please give her this," he responded, handing me a parcel, heavy and thickly wrapped. I put it aside and forgot about it. Some time later we had guests for dinner, so Kate asked me to carry in and carve the roast, which proved to be a large ham with a delicious taste. "Where did you find this fine specimen?" I asked.

"It's a gift from Polly's parents. You remember, she died of leukemia," Kate said. I felt I had been carrying and carving a memorial to the child.

Another time I was summoned to attend a staff conference in Kate's office and on entering noticed an air of suppressed giggling. Janet announced we had received a gift from a patient. Kate displayed a set of black satin sheets, king-size to fit our bed. Ribald remarks proliferated and we promised to report on the utility of the gift. At the weekend the new sheets were spread.

"Jump into bed," Kate instructed, "we'll try them out." I jumped and promptly slithered right across, falling to the floor on her side. Whichever way we tried, we slid disconcertingly all over the bed. The sheets mysteriously disappeared and I concluded that, like many luxuries, they were overrated.

In early summer I was called to deliver a woman who presented at the hospital in labor. She was from Texas, traveling alone through town on the bus. On examining her I could not feel the fetal head and ordered an x-ray, which revealed an anencephalic fetus, lacking a complete skull and all the forebrain. This represents an extreme example of a neural tube defect, manifested in lesser degree in children with spina bifida. I explained the condition to my new patient and answered her questions. The baby was born alive but died within hours. Talking to her afterwards I stressed that it did not appear to be a genetic or hereditary syndrome but that, early in this particular pregnancy, something had interfered with the development of the central nervous system. I assured her that nothing she had done or failed to do had any bearing on the outcome, and tried to assuage her inevitable feelings of guilt and failure.

The second day following delivery I told the nurse, "We can discharge her now."

"Yes, but where to, she has a hole in her jeans and not a nickel in her shoe. We better contact a social worker."

"Today is Friday," I replied. "It will take too long, besides, she's out-of-state and ineligible. Has she any plans?"

"I don't know, she won't open up to me," the RN replied.

I asked my patient if she wanted to leave and where she wanted to go. "I planned to have the—my baby—in Canada," she answered. "I have a friend up there just over the border. I can't face going home yet. I'd like to continue on, rest up, recover my spirits then return to Pecos."

"You're alone aren't you, with little money?"

"Yes, but I have a round-trip Greyhound ticket. I'll be O.K."

"Maybe. I'll find out when the bus leaves Pasco northbound."

This proved to be around midday. "How will you reach Pasco?"

"I don't know, I'll get there somehow."

"I'll be finished here in an hour or so. I'll take you on my way to the office."

She protested but it was arranged. In the car I asked if she had any money. "I've got a ten-spot hidden," she admitted.

"The nurses thought you were busted," I revealed.

"They don't know how to hide things and live rough," she said, and managed a smile. I dropped her at the bus station and, in farewell, she said, "You've been kind. I understand what happened to my baby. I was lucky to meet you. Goodbye."

Just before Labor Day a package arrived for me, postmarked from Texas. It contained no message, but a handsome belt buckle, cowboy style, with my initials on it in heavy shining metal. I took it to the western store, had it fitted to a belt, and bought a new pair of jeans. Now I was correctly dressed for the parade, county fair, and rodeo that enlivened town each fall.

One gift had peculiar repercussions. Notre Dame University invited me to participate in a conference on obstetrics. Following an interesting day my host, a Monsignor, gave me a parcel containing a blue sweatshirt with the Notre Dame name and seal in gold prominently on the front. I thanked him, saying it would be an honor to wear it.

This remark was prophetic but it proved to be too much of an honor. I was wearing it in Boston on a Sunday in the fall when two large men, father and son, surrounded me.

"What happened to Murphy yesterday?" Father asked.

"Mulligan, too," added the son.

I looked puzzled and said, "I don't know."

"That's right, Sweeney doesn't know either," he responded. We all looked sad and parted. Ruminating, I concluded that football was the subject but I knew nothing of the game or the Irish team. In February, again on a Sunday, I was walking on a beach in Florida, wearing the new shirt. A man stopped me. "Ninety-three to ninety-one, close," he said.

"Yes, indeed, very close," I replied cautiously.

"Flanagan was off his game."

"That he was."

"Macnamara should be at center."

"Indeed he should. Goodbye."

One summer evening in Chicago I was out for a stroll and stopped in a tavern, only to find it full of Irish-Americans. A burly man, somewhat unsteady, draped an arm over my sweatshirt exhaling beer fumes over me. "What year were you in South Bend?" he asked.

"Long ago," I replied. "Let me buy you a drink." That done, I downed mine and made a speedy exit. Danny Kaye, I recalled, had found himself in a similar dilemma. Being pursued by the police in London, he dived into the nearest pub to find it completely filled with Irishmen, well into their cups. Instantly transforming himself into a son of Erin's isle, he sang Danny Boy and Kevin Barry, convincing the regulars and the police of his authenticity. Lacking his talent I eventually decided that impersonating a Notre Dame alumnus was dangerous. Now I wear the shirt only in England, where they assume I am French so never talk to me.

One day I saw a patient with advanced ovarian cancer that had spread from the pelvis to the abdomen. I sent her to Seattle, where they confirmed what I feared: that the treatment was palliation and terminal care, for which they returned her to me. I hospitalized her for a spell, then sent her home, and readmitted her as she weakened, then home again. She was a pleasant woman and we became friends. I had developed the custom of calling patients who were confined to home. One afternoon I called and asked, "What are you doing?"

"Sitting in the kitchen, moping."

"That won't do, it's a crisp fall afternoon. I am stuck inside but you needn't be. You're a gardener, go outside and see what you can do." This unsolicited advice was not a success. We next met in the hospital. "How did you do in the garden?" I asked.

"Dreadful, Doctor. I cried. The yard was in such a state, neglected, all weeds, unkempt. I knew that was what it will be like when I'm gone. Bill doesn't care for gardening." While she was sweet, Bill was the reverse. An artisan and a union man, he visited the office frequently, invariably to argue over cost, hospital bills, my fees, what the union insurance would pay and what it would deny. I told him, "We have said repeatedly that we will accept whatever the union pays. As for the hospital, I will cite a different complication at each readmission and the hospital will accept the union payment. You are not helping by arguing with everyone." A few weeks after his wife's death he reappeared at the office on a Saturday morning. "He wants to see you," Janet said.

"What does he want now?"

"I don't know but he isn't waving the union policy as usual. We're busy. See him now, it'll be quicker."

His opening remark surprised me. "Doctor, do you or your wife fish?"

"No, we don't have the patience or the skill."
"One of your children likes fishing maybe?"
"Yes, Nancy, our older daughter. She's nine. She loves it. But I always get the line tangled up and snag the hook."
"How would it be if I took her fishing this afternoon?"
"Fine, but how can you? It's winter. The river's icing over. What's to catch?"
"Plenty, if you know how."
"O.K., I'll call our housekeeper and ask her to dress Nancy warmly and make sandwiches. When will you collect her?"
"Noon and back at four. No food please, I'll fix that." I told him where we lived and so it was arranged.

He took Nancy to the Yakima River on four consecutive Saturdays. The Yakima is a winding stream that traverses the woods and ends in the Columbia. He taught her how to cast, which bait and lure to use. They caught whitefish and other species, some of which Nancy brought home, filleted for Mother to cook. They built a fire and cooked their food. He introduced her to the animals that frequent the riverbank—water rat, otter, beaver—and to the birds and denizens of the wild wood. From her last outing, Nancy returned with a new tackle box full of hooks and paraphernalia, which she now knew how to use. She had a new rod and reel and the knowledge to use them. Best of all, it augmented our reading, for I loved to share the adventures of Ratty, Toad, and Badger, and now she had seen them. This was the best gift we received, and from an unlikely quarter.

I belatedly realized that the fisherman's attitude during his wife's illness was a result of frustration. Like me, he could do nothing against the cancer, could not stem the advancing tide of death, so he vented his anger on the hospital and me.

―――――

Cases are memorable for a variety of reasons—the patient, pathology, circumstances, or outcome. I recall the following case because of the outcome. An old patient returned with her fourth pregnancy and, after an uneventful course, labor started on Thanksgiving Day. To my surprise, I found that the fetus lay crosswise, making it impossible to deliver vaginally. I consulted Ralph, who examined the patient and the x-rays, and we agreed cesarean section was indicated. Kate scrubbed and received the baby and, following discharge, she arranged that the public health nurse make home visits, as was customary for our section patients. This precaution proved pertinent. On Christmas Eve, the patient called me at home, complaining of cramping abdominal pain and nausea, which she ascribed to something she had eaten or drunk. She had waited all day, not wishing to disturb us, but the pain was getting worse. I asked her to meet me at the hospital, where I saw her about 7:00 PM and admitted her. She was ill with fever, an acute abdomen, and peritonitis. The diagnosis puzzled me, for the tenderness was marked in the upper abdomen. The picture did not fit a post-section complication such as pelvic abscess; the timing and location were wrong. I called Guy, my favorite surgeon, and ordered the tests and x-rays he suggested. As he questioned her, then examined her, our concern increased. We sat alone in the deserted hospital lobby, festive with a tree and decorations. He thought the pathology was in the abdomen; but she did not appear to have appendicitis, a bowel obstruction, or a perforated ulcer. He leaned towards acute cholecystitis, an inflammation of the gall bladder, but was not convinced, wondering if she had hepatitis secondary to drugs or alcoholism. He hoped she might respond to medical treatment and inserted a nasogastric tube for suction and decompression of the bowel, filled her with antibiotics intravenously, and decided to observe her overnight. We told her husband of our decision and our reasons.

At 8:00 AM on Christmas morning the patient was unchanged and Guy decided on surgery. Our nurse anesthetist, experienced and competent, arrived and the operation started. We examined the bowel and inspected the gall bladder, liver, and pelvis, which all appeared normal, with no evidence of an abscess. We placed several drains and closed her. The anesthetist stayed with her in the recovery room but she remained intubated, not being able to breathe on her own. The internist was called, but despite all efforts the patient never recovered from the anesthetic, dying about six hours post-op. An autopsy was mandatory, for this was a post-surgical and maternal death. Saddened, puzzled, and dispirited, we returned to our families at the end of a tragic and miserable Christmas Day.

The autopsy revealed no cause for her illness or death.

A year later, Kate, Ralph, Guy, the anesthetist, and I were sued for malpractice. This was the first malpractice case ever in Kennewick, prompting Ralph to remark that when we arrived, he had prophesied we would be trend-setters. The allegations covered everything that had occurred, from the section to her death, and implied a link between the two. Errors of omission and commission were listed.

Our adversary was a malpractice lawyer from Seattle and we were represented by an experienced local trial attorney. Jury selection was protracted, as the plaintiff's counsel was seeking those who were disgruntled with life in general and doctors in particular. His first question was, "Do you have a prejudice towards or against any of these doctors?"

The first respondent answered, "No, but I am absolutely sure Dr.___ (naming Guy) could not possibly do anything wrong," a sentiment with which I concurred. This prospective juror was rejected. Immediately the proceedings were underway the judge inquired if Kate was accused of negligence, for the baby was alive and well, or was she present merely because of our partnership. Hearing the latter was the case, he excused her from further attendance. Our adversary provided four expert witnesses from California; an obstetrician, surgeon, anesthesiologist, and internist, who articulated a list of our faults in these areas. Our defender questioned them in simple terms, assuming no medical knowledge himself. He asked them to point to one particular error, one that resulted directly in her death, and to give a cause of death. This proved difficult to do—even, as he pointed out, with the benefit of hindsight. As the experts dissembled, the judge became irritable, insisting they answer the two simple questions clearly. The consequence was that four different errors and causes of death were cited.

We presented no experts, just two local practitioners. The public health RN, by means of her record and recollections, established that there was no infection in the mother during the month following her delivery. This exonerated the section as a contributor to her death. Our second witness was the pathologist who performed the autopsy. He proved a formidable advocate for us, for he viewed the plaintiff's counsel and experts as questioning his competence as well as ours. If he could not assign a specific cause of death, who were these interlopers so to presume? Cross-examining him was a losing proposition as his replies were forthright, brief yet lucid, attributes the judge admired. After a week of testimony and closing arguments, during which our counsel pointed out that four experts had reached four different conclusions as to the cause of death and that the pathologist, the person best qualified to make a determination, had been uncertain, the jury retired. After a brief deliberation, they entered a unanimous verdict for the defense and our ordeal ended.

I was culpable in one instance, but no suit resulted. I was about to deliver a patient, the second one that night, to whom I had promised a saddle block, a procedure I performed regularly. This provides complete pain relief in the pelvis, and is suitable for a woman having her first baby. The packs containing the drug, needle and drape were kept in the delivery room but when I asked the nurse for one, she replied, "You've already used the only one we had. I haven't had time to prepare another."

"O.K., run to the OR and get one of their spinal packs, quickly, or we'll be too late," I said. I then sat the patient up on the edge of the delivery table with her feet on a stool and her back arched, her head on my shoulder. The nurse returned, breathless, and took my place. I quickly opened the pack, prepped the patient's back, placed the drapes, cracked open the glass vial, and filled the syringe with the entire contents, exactly as I always did. I took the long spinal needle and felt her back, which was well flexed, for she was young and having her first baby. The intervertebral space was easy to locate and I guided the needle in, slick as a whistle. The spinal fluid dripped out and I slowly injected the contents of the syringe in the usual way. Then we replaced her on the table, re-draped her for delivery, and I took a smaller needle and tapped the skin of her thigh with it, asking, "Is this sharp or dull? Tell me when you feel it sharp."

She replied "Dull, dull," as I tapped her on the abdomen, higher than usual. Suddenly, I remembered that the vials in the OR packs contained twice as much anesthetic agent as those in the delivery room. They were the same size, looked exactly the same, and contained the identical volume, but the concentration was twice as strong. I jumped up from the stool and turned the crank on the table, raising her head and dropping her feet in an attempt to prevent the anesthetic from rising any higher in the spinal canal and paralyzing her breathing. The nurse was unwrapping the forceps for me to deliver the baby. I whispered, "Call Roy (our nurse anesthetist) in here stat."

"Why? I've never seen you do it slicker, Dead Eye Dick."

"Go get him now, I'll explain later, hurry."

The baby was fine but it took Roy two hours of skillful support of her respiration before the mother was out of danger. After this we changed the vials, marked each distinctively, and took every precaution to prevent a repetition. My patient was delighted with the outcome and told me, "I never felt anything, thank you."

Another time I made the gynecologist's classic mistake: I did not consider causes outside the pelvis. I did not look at the whole patient. I failed to think the case over deeply and took no consult before scheduling surgery. In mitigation, I plead I was obliging a friend, whose wife was my patient. But this is no excuse, for I was experienced in treating friends' wives, doctors' wives, nurses, and others whom I knew well.

Jenny, a mother of five, was in her forties, married to Ted, a lawyer. They were among the few close friends we had who were not doctors and so especially prized. Frequently we had dinner at their home or at the club.

Ted explained to me, "Jenny is always bleeding, not much, starting and stopping, no pattern to it. She says it's the menopause and she'll get over it, but I'm worried. She won't see her GP but she might go to you."

I examined her, took a cervical smear, and admitted her for a D&C, which showed no cancer. I hoped the D&C might stop the bleeding, but was disappointed. Ted called and said, "I understand Jenny does not have cancer, which is a relief, but she's no better; in fact, worse. You know the blood is coming from the uterus. Can't you do something about it, something permanent? We don't want any more children."

I performed a hysterectomy, which appeared uneventful, but the anesthetist fussed, unusual for him, and kept her in the recovery room longer than normal.

Late that evening, the ward called me at home. "Your post-op is behaving strangely. She's restless. She seems apprehensive. She's plucking at the sheets and trying to pull the IV out." As I drove to the hospital, I thought, "It can't be, not in Jenny."

Her large private room was in shadow, with only one lamp lit. The bed was near the window. As I entered, Jenny said, "Close the door! They'll get in. Look, they're running up the drapes."

There was the diagnosis, running up the drapes, and I had missed it stone cold, no excuses. I had seen plenty of cases, but in London, Baltimore and especially in Brooklyn, not in a private room in the wife of one of the prominent men in the TriCities and, sadly, in a woman who was our close friend. Delirium tremens is a serious complication of alcoholism. Patients with the DTs are difficult to manage. They pull the dressings off, the IVs out, shout and thrash about. They need restraints and sedation. Their medical complications are severe and life-threatening. Jenny was discharged alive but died in three months from cirrhosis.

Hindsight was clear. The uterine bleeding was due to liver failure. She was a hidden alcoholic but Ted was complicit, he had to be. Jenny had an old beat-up car full of dents. We thought they used it for rough hauling and trips into the hills where they didn't want to take Ted's Cadillac, which she never drove. She drank no alcohol in our company, which was always in the evening. Jenny drank vodka all day at home, bought clandestinely in the poorest part of Pasco. She slept, then sobered up for her evenings out. She had deceived me completely.

I operated on an elderly lady in Pasco. I visited the evening prior to surgery and found her serene. The operation was uneventful. The OR and recovery room were on the top floor and had a good view of a Pasco landmark, a large water tower. Due to a muddle over which bed she should have after surgery, she was held in the recovery room longer than usual, watched by an aide who had the radio playing gospel music.

The next morning, I visited her and said the operation had gone well and I was optimistic for an early discharge and complete recovery.

"How do you feel?" I enquired.

"Disappointed. My spirits are down. My hopes are gone," she answered.

"But why?" I asked.

"When I woke I couldn't see but I could hear the holy music playing and the angels singing," she responded fervently, "and I thought, Lord be praised, I'm in heaven as I long to be. But when I opened my eyes, I saw the water tower and knew I was still in Pasco."

Waldo was a drug salesman and a friend. Indefatigable as a pitch man for SMA, a milk formula for babies, he had one weakness, the bottle.

One evening I found him despondent in his motel room.

"What's wrong, Waldo? Having trouble making the quota this month?" I asked.

"No, Dick, no worse than usual," he replied pushing the Scotch, ice, and glass towards me, "but I had a dreadful experience this morning."

"Relax, Waldo. Unburden."

"Yesterday was Monday," he said morosely," and you're right, I was worrying about the quota. This is the last week of the month. So, last night, up in Yakima, I will admit I had a drop too much. Felt terrible this morning, couldn't touch breakfast, so I got on the road and resolved I would first visit that woman GP up the valley. Know her?"

"Vaguely. Big and hearty, right? A tough customer, I'd guess."

"Right. I gave her the pitch and she asked, 'Is it palatable?'"

"SMA! Palatable, doctor? Certainly! It's nutritious and delicious,' I responded."

"Make us two glasses full then" she bellowed at me. "It'll set us up for the morning.'"

Reliving the ordeal shook Waldo, so he replenished our glasses. SMA was no doubt irresistible to infants every hour of the twenty-four, but not necessarily to adults. Waldo resumed.

"Her nurse produced two damn great glasses and I made it up and carried them back to her office. She grabbed hers and cried, 'Down the hatch' and swallowed the lot, almost in one gulp, then stared at me." He paused. "I've given everything for the company, Dick. Always put it first."

"I know, Waldo, you're the best in the business. But this?"

"Exactly. The supreme sacrifice. I dared not hesitate, just closed my eyes and slugged it down. God knows how. Managed to keep my dignity and made it to the parking lot before I…"

"Waldo, please spare us both the details. Let's have another."

One of the things that drew me to obstetrics was excitement, for emergencies are frequent. In the middle of a busy afternoon the front office interrupted me. "There's an excited woman calling. I can't understand her but I think it's an emergency. Will you take it?"

"Yes, put her on." I cannot comprehend a word of any foreign tongue but I thought, from my Brooklyn days, this is Spanish. I shouted at Janet, "Can Bernie speak Spanish?"

"A bit. She was brought up in L.A."

"O.K., switch this call to her. Careful, don't lose it."

In a minute Bernie came on to say, "She's calling from Pasco and I'm pretty sure describing a pregnant woman bleeding and collapsed in the toilet, and she said the name of Alice [wife of Guy, my special surgeon]. I've got her on hold."

"Right, tell the caller the ambulance is coming." Then, to Janet, "Send the ambulance to Guy's house, stat. Instruct them to take her to Pasco Hospital. Then call delivery there and alert them that we'll be doing an emergency section." I collected her chart, then told Kate, "I'm going to Pasco now. I figure she has a previa [bleeding from a low-lying placenta] or possibly an abruption [premature separation of the placenta]. In either case we'll probably do a section. I'll call you after I have seen her."

She was due in seven or eight weeks. The sudden severe bleed was surprising, for the pregnancy had been uneventful. There had been no complications such as an early bleed, which often occurs in previa. This was her fifth pregnancy and the previous four had been normal. As I drove across the river I recalled her husband was away at a meeting in Seattle. The patient was conscious on arrival but the medics reported finding her collapsed in the bathroom, having suffered a large blood loss. They had revived her and started an IV. She had bright red bleeding, a soft belly and no pain, which indicated a previa and heralded a better prognosis for the fetus, which would have been dead had this been abruption. The fetus felt small and the heart rate was rapid. The patient was concerned first for her husband, and said, "Please don't call Guy. He can't help now. If he rushes back he may have an accident on the road."

"I promise he won't know until you are both O.K.," I replied, going on to explain that due to the rate and amount of bleeding, early delivery was essential. This meant section, since labor had not started and could not be expected due to the prematurity. I did not add, for she knew, that the outlook for her baby was uncertain because of blood loss and consequent deprivation of fetal circulation, poorly sustained by a premature. I was not worried about the mother, for she was a common blood group of which there was an adequate supply. The surgery was uneventful but the baby had seventy-two hours of difficulty breathing and she remained hospitalized until she had attained five pounds.

This emergency resolved happily but, as years passed and cases accumulated, the excitement which I had enjoyed began to take a toll.

We sought partners, without success. Being on call perpetually was difficult to withstand, although we got used to it. A summons from a doctor or the hospital inevitably took precedence over everything, with no exception. The result was that one of us, at random, was liable to leave precipitously for the hospital. With obstetrical complications involving the fetus, we were both called. When this occurred at night and we had only one child, Kate would take our daughter to the hospital. Later, when we had several, the hospital would send an aide to our home at night until one of us returned. Despite this consideration, and that of our colleagues and patients, the strain continued.

It was late 1967 when I started to twitch. My right eye, the right side of my face, and my right hand were affected. At first, it occurred only at night when I received a call from a doctor asking me to come to the hospital for a difficult delivery. I would recover by the time I had dressed, and my work was unaffected. Later, I twitched whenever faced by an emergency, whatever the cause.

One evening in the summer of 1968, Kate had a surprise for me, saying, "I have done your thing for eleven years, worked in the practice, had the children and enjoyed it. But I don't intend to spend the rest of my life here, doing the same thing over and over. I'm thirty-seven and need a change. I have to force the issue or I'll be stuck. You enjoy your role here. You've refused two good jobs, one with Syntex and one in Portland. Despite what you may promise, the reality is that you will stay here doing hysterectomies and delivering babies. Don't you ever get bored? Surely there's only a certain number of ways a baby can come into the world?"

"That's true, my love."

"To make it easier for you, I've made a decision and accepted a position as assistant professor at a medical school. They want me after Labor Day for the new academic year but I could string them along until January. But that's it. It would give you time to look around if you decide to come with us."

I was astonished that she had, in secret, negotiated a contract. She had told me she was going to a pediatric meeting, which had been true except that it was with her prospective employer. Giving me the choice of remaining in Kennewick was a mark of equality. I had left her to go to

Hopkins, saying, "Please come and join me in America, but you are free to remain in England." Now, she had made me a similar proposition. She intended to develop her career, and I realized I must do the same.

The last farewell I said was to Ralph, who responded characteristically.

"Ralph, I've come to say goodbye. I'm sorry to be leaving."

"No, you're not, you're glad, and I understand why."

"I've learned a lot from you and enjoyed working with you immensely. We'll always be friends."

"No, we won't. Friendships like ours are born of shared times, tasks, and interests. You are moving on and will face new concerns and make new friends. I wish you well. Goodbye."

So began the next chapter in our lives.

About the Author

Dr. Morton left his practice in Washington State in 1968, at age 44. Following three years of study at UCLA, he returned to Baltimore and taught at the University of Maryland School of Medicine and at The Johns Hopkins University School of Public Health. In 1978 he moved to New York, becoming Medical Director of the March of Dimes Birth Defects Foundation, and taught at the Albert Einstein College of Medicine. He and his wife Kate are now retired and live in Florida during the winter and England in the summer.

To order a copy of this book, call 1-800-253-0900.